Coffee on 2nd Street

The true story of a man's life and
his victorious battle with Alzheimer's

Dr. Steve Norby
Mary Ann Shires Montgomery

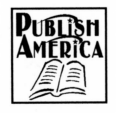

PublishAmerica
Baltimore

First printing

ISBN: 1-4137-1050-6
PUBLISHED BY PUBLISHAMERICA, LLLP
www.publishamerica.com
Baltimore

Printed in the United States of America

For Tom and Rennie...

ACKNOWLEDGEMENTS

Special thanks to Dean Mathews for the use of Rennie's family chronicles. Also to Taproots Press for permission to publish Tom's poetry.

Thanks to Laurin Sydney and Nicole von Ruden for the words of encouragement, and to Elizabeth Aebischer for the rushed and last minute editing.

We would also like to acknowledge the lives of the many scientists through whose dedication and personal sacrifice we have a greater understanding of the human mind.

Preface

From The Long Good Night

I meant to say I love you all the times I should,
all the drear sad times you needed that to hold –
Not half as much as I planned to say,
nor a hundredth what would keep at bay
the deranged dragons in the dark
for one more night....
If I could not bear to part with the storm of you
how much should I have mourned each raindrop
as it fell away....

Dr. O. Thomas Law

The above poem is a glimpse into the passion and depth of love one person can hold for another. Fighting for nearly a decade to prevent the dementia that accompanies Alzheimer's, Dr. O. Thomas Law wrote many such poems. It is a fight that has not *always* been successful, for there have been long nights of vigil where Rennie lay comatose on the floor, and only an eyedropper with liquid nutrient, placed lovingly between her lips – sometimes stretching into hours or even days – only that, could bring her back. When all others had given up hope, a short, heavy, bearded old college professor kneels beside his fallen mate through the dark night. A form of alchemy is taking place; it is the admixture of one of the most brilliant scientific minds ever to exist, combined with a love beyond reason.

One drop at a time, he retrieves his wife. One caress at a time, she is returned from the abyss, and when she revives, it is as if the episode never took place for her. She awakens, then embraces Tom. Weak, she is weak, but alive and vital once again. Her memory returns, complete with the recollection of passion she holds for this man – the passion that compelled her to leave teaching and sail for countless years on a small boat in the Sea of Cortez; a form of honeymoon that never ended.

Despite the victory, it takes a toll on Tom, for in truth, he had said goodbye sometime during the night. When she is safe and resting, he finds expression on the keyboard of his computer. Shut down, for the moment, are the complex formulas, nutrients and cofactors that he uses to keep her alive. The intellectual side of his mind stops, and the suppressed emotions pour out on pages.

He laments his weakness;
"Can you forgive me if sometimes it was all I could do
to keep you safe one more time?
Sometimes it seemed the whole of life
was not just dying.
All I might have done groans in the wind now
and blows away…
…whispers of adieu."

To understand Dr. O. Thomas Law is to attempt to understand two people at once. There is a scientist. He unraveled the secrets of the brain via brilliant and revolutionary experiments. He uncovered the neural pathways that for a large part determine our behavior, and more or less, he proved that our behavior is driven by basic and primal motives. This is the Tom that taught in medical schools and uprooted many antiquated theories. To listen to him lecture or speak is to be humbled - if you ever had any misconceptions that Mankind is a quantum leap ahead of other species in certain ways.

We are not, it seems, all that different.

And yet, there is the other part of him. This is the part that is revealed through actions; the passion and dedication he has to his wife – the passion and love he holds for all creation.

As I worked through the information and his teachings, I initially fell victim to despair. Personally, I needed the security of safe boundaries in my beliefs. I required the comfort that walls and limitations can provide. But Tom is not about limitations, and his devastating logic breaks through barriers like tissue paper. In spite of my academic background, I often found that I needed to take his revelations in measured doses.

When I complained to Tom about this and expressed the challenges I was facing in letting go of my closely-guarded beliefs, he sympathized and commented, "Quite so. And to have the courage to do so is most commendable. I know the pressures. One can die from them. It's possible to go beyond that position though. And that becomes very hard to explain. Succinctly but inadequately one passes to a place in the mind where they are no longer relevant, no longer meaningful. One has gone beyond the question of faith and immortality to a place where they are utterly without meaning."

Later still I asked him, in a fit of trying to find meaning in my life, "So how do you reconcile our plight with a sense of grace? Or, in other words, is there anything about being human that is worth a damn? If we are a 'mechanism' of genetic programming, it is useful for suspending judgment, but not much use in offering value to our existence. We *need* the value."

Tom responded, "Look *up,* Steve, look at the moon. There are *human* footprints there. No other living thing could even aspire to that glory … only a struggle that Olympic is worthy of us… the moon will always be there to remind us of what we can be."

Reaching further into Tom's personal philosophies, I read his poem, *The Third Eye*, which in his notes he defines as follows; "…it is with this eye that we see those things to which our ordinary consciousness is blind. It is also with our third eye that we envision The Divine Presence."

This is the life story of Dr. O. Thomas Law, or rather, it is the story of the two people inside of him. The first, a scientist. Calculating, analytical, and ready at any time to levy devastating logic on our frail philosophies. The second, a sensitive and hopeless romantic, a person whose depth and compassion defy logical explanation - a person who perceives a place; *"…where with an endless lever of light, you can pry the seams of the Universe apart."*

Dr. Steve Norby

Preface by author Mary Ann Shires Montgomery.

When my Dentist son approached me to ask if I'd like to co-author a biography about one of his patients, Dr. O. Tom Law, I quickly said, 'Sure I would!' However, I would be less than honest if I didn't admit that it wasn't for any other reason than the mere fact that my son is one of my favorite people in the entire world. Why wouldn't I want to spend some quality time with him and well, if a good biography came out of it, then the time would be well spent. I was involved in writing my 3rd book and a children's book, co-authored with my daughter, that were well under way to being published. I took it all as a good omen.

What I wasn't prepared for was the actuality of Dr. Tom and Our Wren, as we now lovingly call them. I should have known when I first looked into the swimming blueness and depth of Tom's eyes – full of both accepted sadness and unabashed love and then Rennie's big, brown adoring eyes that are so full of compassion and caring for everyone – especially Tom. It is so very obvious they are special that I immediately understood my son's desire and determination to write their life story, and they, very quickly, became the object of my wholehearted attention.

I remembered them vaguely in years past, riding up to my son's dental office on their motorcycle. Then later after their appointments, watching them climb back on the motorcycle, Tom's wild, white hair untucked under his helmet and Rennie's long braids undulating sinuously down her back as they rode off down the road. I especially remembered my son's delight when he knew Tom had an appointment on any given day. They spoke the same language and Steve greatly admired and enjoyed Tom's brilliant mind.

It wasn't until some time later that I realized what Tom and Rennie had been going through all those many years. In a small town like ours, word eventually gets around and ultimately, everyone knows and wants to help in their own way.

But sometimes the struggle is so personal that it is only shared when desperation sets in along with reality. Alzheimers is that sort of disease; that's what Tom faced with his beloved Rennie.

From the depths of his heart, and in his grief, this scientist wrote unimaginable poetry - too extraordinary to believe. And, through it all, he nurtured, cared for and eventually arrested the disease in Rennie.

Today she is a viable lady, full of life and love and most of all, many, many memories. And the good news is, they are making more of those memories and sharing them with all of us.

Their love still physically shows with a smile and the look in their eyes as they glance at one another. They are an inspiration to all of us that love really doesn't fade away with the passing of years. If anything, it is enhanced – improved like fine wine – with age and understanding.

But what makes a person like Tom make the choice to see this situation through for Rennie? What is inside this brilliant scientist that filled him with so much love and determination that he gave up his own free will – even his life – to live under the most strenuous and horrific circumstances. He held fast even when he didn't really see any hope for the future.

The selfless love that Tom exhibited, and indeed still does, for Rennie in her time of desperate need is so admirable that it is almost overwhelming. A love like theirs is a rarity in our world and certainly their wonderful story is deserving of being shared. By allowing us a glimpse into their lives, we are able to realize there is hope, and hope is the one enduring quality and glimmer of that illusive dream that keeps us all going.

In the minds of the authors, (and certainly Rennie's), Tom is surely a hero of the finest kind and has the essential qualities that we all admire so much in a human being. His gentle and considerate nature is balanced by his splendid mind and unwavering determination as exhibited by his life story herein.

The lasting and wonderful thing about this love story is that it is true and therefore, even more exhilarating for all of us.

I feel privileged to know and write about O. Tom Law and Rennie Clark Law - privileged to have the opportunity to enjoy them and call them friends. I breathe in their knowledge, trust of life and love deep into my soul—the admixture that they exhibit - and it gives me courage in a sometimes troubled world.

We need people like the Laws to come into and touch our lives once in awhile. It keeps us balanced and gives us the ability to experience life and love and to become deeply and excessively involved with something subjectively felt as pleasant, stimulating and most of all, loving.

And perhaps through it all, we are left with a sense of hope that there is more to and for all of us than just existing.

Now, I know and understand why my son felt such a calling to write this book.

We hope you enjoy it.

Mary Ann Shires Montgomery

Chapter One

Botticelli's Angel

You sought to be this work,
To haunt this vivid mirror,
To stick the slip of time
And splatter stops of black and chrome
In a frame of mind.

I will paint you lying on your side
Eyes closed, holding a ghost.
I will paint you lying on your back,
Eyes wide open, heels locked about life.
I will paint you with an eyelash for a brush
On the silver canvas of the moon.
On your knees I will paint you
With your hands around a butterfly.
Monarch and mate, tongue and thigh.
I will paint you standing straight
Where your shadows fill the spaces
Spread between the shrinking sparks
Over the toothed texture of the awful truth.
When I am done, sketched the last dark line,
I will scrape the palette clean again
And you and I shall hang it high
On the western wall of the world.

By O. Tom Law

"It's the bottom of the hill love...rest now."

Tom holds his hand up in front of his face, but even then he can barely see his fingers in the early evening twilight.

Finger fog. Elongated whiffs slip sideways, touching everything in their way in cooperation with the soft breeze, making the pier barely visible. The dense fog moves almost rhythmically now as its fine particles continue to dance just beyond his focused vision. It winds in, around, over and under the wooden rails that outline the pier.

It is that kind of fog and it's rolling in across the water and off the Back Bay, pouring onto 2nd street and beyond. It tumbles and rolled over itself only to edge ever further onto the shore and upward across the street. Thick and then thinner, the fingers of fog crept onshore cooling and washing all the air in its path – natures own air conditioning, courtesy of the blue Pacific Ocean.

It is five p.m. and already there is a hint of twilight as Tom and Rennie take their usual seats at the little wooden table provided by the Coffee n' Things coffeehouse. None of their friends are present this evening, so there might not be any poetry shared. It didn't matter, perhaps they would turn up later. Possibly, Tom thought, there would be an audience of friends later on for his latest sonnet.

Minnie, their little Corgi, curled up under the table in her usual spot. Her luminous, brown eyes scan the rough concrete for any sign of scraps, and then returned to Tom and Rennie in hopeful anticipation of a snack. The tables outside are placed with this dual purpose in mind. That way, all the usual coffee drinkers with dogs can walk them to the coffeehouse and not have to leave them tied outside - or, worse yet – (in the minds of the proprietors) - not bring them at all.

Everyone that lives here knows it is a "dog" town. A haven for retirees, Baywood Park also has its contingent of professionals. The casual ambience, along with the moderate climate attracts artists, couples, recluses and the occasional intellectual as well.

Situated snugly on the water and protruding into the estuary, Baywood is more an extension of Morro Bay than it is a unique geographic entity. But don't try to tell that to the people that live here, as they consider the area as different from Morro Bay as the moon is from the sun.

It used to be nothing more than an isolated pile of sand years ago. During the 2nd World War, tanks from Camp San Luis practiced running over the dunes that make up the area. There was even a small Coast Guard base at the far end of the Bay complete with horses and dogs. Since there was not a second water outlet (and to this day it remains the same), it was considered secure from any surprise attack.

It was, and still is, an orderly town that provides conditions that make for comfort and security for the people that live there. Now, those same dunes afford beautiful views of the ocean and in the evening, the flickering lights of the towns to the north with a halo of light from San Luis Obispo a few miles to the southeast.

Because of its proximity to the ocean, property values have gone steadily up over the last several decades. What, years ago, was just a little fishing village, a place for people from the central valley to come to get out of the heat in the summer and maybe fish a little, has finally come into its own.

Situated gently on the central coast of California, Baywood has everything from wonderful weather to the availability and desirability of being about halfway between Santa Barbara and Monterey. It is a small town in numbers, surrounded by ocean and state parks, and the people that live there would just as soon keep it that way.

The Bay itself, barely a rock's throw from where Tom and Rennie are sitting, is separated by a large sand spit from the Pacific Ocean and therefore is protected from the most severe storms. However, as the valleys of the central coast heat up, fog is drawn in from the ocean and so summer weather - all six weeks of it - is usually enjoyed in the fall months. That's when the valley cools down and Mother Nature doesn't bother sending in the cooling fog.

It's late September and the shorter days, with the fine display of uncommonly colored sunsets, are a welcome sight when the evenings are clear.

Both Tom and Rennie stare at the incoming wisps of fog, arriving as if carried by the tide – a tide that silently and gently takes a further bite out of the sandy mud at the shoreline. Rennie smiles as Tom takes her hand in his and asks if she's warm enough in her jacket.

"Oh, yes. I'm just fine."

Two mugs of hot coffee are placed in front of them with just a smile and a nod from the waiter. He knows them well, as they are here just about everyday and have been for several years. They always arrive about this time. They come and watch the sunset as it dips behind the sandspit. Some of the time, they enjoy their coffee and conversation with friends and then later, they walk the several blocks back to their home for dinner.

It seems to the waiter that there is no other purpose to their perennial visits, and yet, unbeknownst to him, there is deep significance and meaning to this migratory return.

The little Corgi sits up and nudges Rennie's leg - acknowledging the delivery of the expected coffee and hoping for a treat.

They slowly sip their coffee in silence staring at the ever-changing scene across the water. Lights are flickering on now, one by one, on the small peninsula across the Bay and as the fog settles in, the surrealistic picture it paints is beautiful.

"Fireflies, Rennie," Tom says, "The lights flash like the fireflies in Mexico. Do you remember them?"

"Yes," she replies, "Yes, like in Tecalpan, I remember...they were beautiful."

Tom stares back out over the water and his thoughts are, as always, of Rennie. He thinks how happy he is that she is able to answer him in this manner. It still amazes even him. If he were to describe her to someone - anyone - he would describe her first as a lady. A gentle, intelligent and beautiful lady, even in her eighty-seventh year.

As he steals a sidelong glance at her silhouette, so familiar even in the fading twilight, he is struck by the awesome dichotomy of the last several years they have survived and conquered. Yes, conquered would be the right and only fitting word.

The pungent smell of the Bay seems to arrive with the fog. It lightly touches their noses with its sharp and stimulating odor and appropriately combines with the silence of the impending twilight.

With the tantalizing smell of fresh-brewed coffee, Tom's mind inadvertently flashes back to the most frightening scene of his life. It floods him with horrible images.

Let it lie. Don't bring it up again.
It never comes to much,
And yet it never lets us be.

Eight bells and nothing's well.

I suppose it must come up again
Between us,
Bounding out of the fresh ground
And shoving us out of the way
With its restless stir.

It was 4 a.m. in the morning when it happened. Rennie was one of the one in a hundred Alzheimer's patients that became ever more violent with time. In her despair and depression, she had become suicidal and it seemed that her attempts became more and more violent as time progressed. As a matter of fact, so did she.

Alzheimer's is insidious and insistently compels your attention. It comes on, seemingly, faster and faster until it is just there - staring everyone in the face - and you are left wondering how and exactly when it happened.

Rennie had been attempting suicide by every means possible to her. She slashed her wrists, but not enough to really do any permanent damage. She harangued and harassed Tom, trying to get him to help her die - to put her out of her endless misery and to help her leave this world so she wouldn't have to go through what she knew to be the ultimate end with Alzheimer's.

It had gone on this time for at least 48 endless hours. Neither of them had slept during that time and they were both exhausted, mentally and physically. Finally, in a vain attempt to just get away from her for a moment, Tom went outside intending to get some fresh air to clear his mind - to take a brief walk down the street. It was about 3 a.m. then and just as he reached the pavement of the road, Rennie flung the front door open, ran out and literally chased him down the street, screaming and yelling. The fact that he had walked away and out the door was enough to set her off again. He was sure the neighbors would call the police so he gave up and hurriedly went back into the house.

It was at that time, and in his desperation, that he finally called the suicide hotline and had them to talk with her. That gave him a moment's peace, but

17

there was no prospect of hope by then. He remembered shouting, "Dammit, if you are going to kill yourself, then do it right and get it over with! Here, look at this!" He held his .44 caliber, muzzle-loading revolver that hangs above his desk in his hand. It is always loaded - which is to say that there is powder, patch and ball (round ball – 1860 vintage) in every cylinder. But, it can't be fired until a cap is placed, outside, on the nipple.

Tom started to offer it to her, knowing it couldn't possibly be fired, but knowing that she didn't know that. He thought to call her bluff without placing her in any real danger, but he couldn't get her attention away from the suicide hotline. So, in his own bleak despair, it occurred to him, what the hell, why not…demonstrate. Tom suddenly felt the overwhelming burden of months of pain tumble over him like an obscure veil of cobwebs. He put a cap on one cylinder, spun it, put the gun in his mouth and pulled the trigger. Click. Spun the cylinder. Click again. Four times. Four times nothing. With the fourth spin and click, the sheriff's car pulled into their driveway. The suicide hotline had heard him in the background and called them…at least that was what he assumed - and it was over.

His mind back in the present now with the fog surrounding them, Tom looks at Rennie. Her familiar face, her tall body wrapped tightly against the cool of the evening – a body so sweetly familiar. The fog is still thick and water continually drips from the branches of the large, old cedar trees. The shore has become hard to see even from such a short distance although they can hear the water lapping against the dock. His heart fills with an overwhelming rush of love for Rennie as he looks at her and remembers how far she has come from that fateful night. It has been a struggle for both of them. Are we the same two people that went through those trying, horrible times? Hard to believe we did. Even harder to believe he actually felt so distraught he had attempted suicide in order to show her how to do it - even though that wasn't the real reason.

They finished their coffee and stood up to leave. Minnie danced her way around the table not wanting to be left behind.

Tom thought, as he gently took Rennie's hand, "We have come a long way from those awful times. Such a very long way to get to this point. I can't help but wonder how much further we can go…"

Before the shadows grow too tall…

You have so far to go,
Miles of desert from one vineyard to the next:
Even a poor wine will wet the wasteland
And better itself with age.
Take this bottle of spring and harvest past,
Stoppered for the dry days. A gift to you.
To warm the mind and wet the throat
And savor in the sandy days...

Chapter Two

"I don't understand this cycle of life and death," Steve told Tom, "I don't understand the meaning of it all..."

Tom Law sat quietly in his chair. He shifted his weight a little to alleviate his continuous pain, then regarded his former dentist with stark, blue eyes, "You're asking if there is more to the rose than birth and death, but for the rose, isn't that enough? Look, as the blossom fades and darkens into dust, it becomes something else. It's not lost. Neither is the beauty. It's reborn. And yes, that's it. Not the same blossom, but its message. The message it received the previous season, passed on by every blossom and seed in its lineage for billions of years, honing and polishing the message of perfection of seed and blossom. The message is reborn each generation, and that is why there are seeds and blossoms, men, women and children - so that the message will be passed on. Nothing else – anything more would be a burden to the efficiency of the transmission. No hulks, no shells, no mortal coils – just information. And in the process, the information itself becomes changed. That's the way the phenomenon begins and ultimately, ends."

Dr. Tom sat back in his chair, took another swallow of his coffee and smiled.

It was dreary and trying to rain that July night in 1925 when O. Tom Law was forced into this world. Summer in West Virginia was hot and humid with thunderstorms and given to rain at any time. Tom's mother, Genevieve Kate Roberts, entered the Presbyterian Hospital in Clarksburg at about three a.m. Tom's dad drove her to the hospital and after making sure she was securely in the proper care of the night nurse, he left.

"No need for me to hang around is there, Berbie? Work to do on the farm and all." And with a jaunty little tap of his cap, he was off and gone. She didn't expect more.

She struggled through her labor, comforted only by the nurses until a calm peacefulness enveloped her. The nurses noticed it each in their own way and smiled - they recognized the signs. They had been down that road a time or two before.

O. Tom Law was born without much fuss and his mother, with perspiration dripping from her tired face, cradled her son in her arms and smiled as she looked into his eyes. She knew instinctively without thinking about it, that theirs would grow into a special relationship. Tears streamed down her cheeks and with a catch in her throat she softly whispered to him, "It'll be alright, my baby – it will all be all right in the end."

She knew his life would be a difficult one and committed herself to helping him as best she could. She never forgot that first tender look between mother and son in the years that followed and as she predicted, theirs was always a special relationship.

As the nurses put Tom back into a little newborn crib, he had to crane his neck to look back at his mother. He continued to stare in her direction as the nurses cleaned and wrapped him then gently placed the crib nearby. He looked at his mother and fixed his blue eyes on her as if to say, "I finally made it. I'm here."

Tom was the third and last child to be born into the Law family that made their home about 20 miles from Clarksburg. It was during the Great Depression years and they lived on 80 acres of hill farm, until some years later when they were able to take over and run the Robert's Hardware store in Clarksburg. Farming was difficult, but at least it supplied a family with food. Later they were able to move off the farm and closer into town where there were other families, but by that time, all the boys were considerably older. They had a lonely life until then.

The family was considered small by normal Appalachian standards. Tom's dad had nine brothers and sisters – a "normal" sized family. Tom's grandparents, Lewis and Adaline Law were married in 1879 in Harrison County, West Virginia. They lived in Two Lick and then Good Hope until Lewis' father, James S. Law, a captain in the Union Army during the Civil War, gave Lewis and Adaline 200 acres. Eventually they used the timber from their land to build a thirteen room two-story house that, among other attributes, included two stairwells and thirteen fireplaces, complete with cellar. The home stood proudly for many years and the sawdust house, used for ice storage, is still standing.

Homesteading, farming or sharecropping, the pioneers of those days needed lots of children to help with the work and hopefully, some of them would stay with the family when they grew up.

Often, however, this was not to be the case. The children growing up in Appalachia suspected there was a better life away from the farm, but by leaving, they suffered severe admonishments by their parents. Sacrifices had been made in raising them, they were reminded, and the obligation that they were to stay around and help the aging generation was understood at a very young age.

The Law family lived on just such a farm. They raised cows, sheep, pigs and chickens and farmed the bottomland providing almost everything they needed to survive. Tom's mother canned, cooked, sewed and tended her garden and apple orchid – just as most women of her generation did. Tom's dad worked the land, planting the crops and tending the outbuildings, but it took the whole family to provide enough food for the harsh winters and still have money left over to buy seed for the next year's crops and necessities. It was a hard enough life for adults and even more difficult for the three boys. Endless days of work left little time to be children and play was out of the question.

Tom's father was relentless to the point of being almost brutal when it came to working the boys. He demanded and expected more of them than they were sometimes capable of giving and by so doing, stripped them of any dignity by his lack of understanding or praise. Tom's main job was tending the cows – a formidable task at any time, but especially so when you are very young and not particularly tall. Yet tending the cows was just the beginning of his chores and as he grew, so did the amount of work his father required of him. When his two older brothers were in school, Tom worked twice as hard just trying to compensate for their absence. At least there was never time for fights or arguments with his siblings----they were never allowed any free time and would have been too tired regardless.

Tom thought about life at a very early age. As he observed his own family, each one in their turn, he knew there must be another way to live and he couldn't understand why his parents would purposely choose this one. But he would not have dared ask his dad and when he mentioned it to his mother, she just wistfully smiled and said that she agreed with him – there had to be several other ways to live and that he should think about it when he got older. He wondered why she hadn't thought of a way herself, but he didn't dare ask. It all made him sad, and in his young mind he began to attribute the harshness of their lives as somehow causing the same painful and distressing severity and meanness in his dad.

He was contemplating these thoughts one day while chopping wood and he realized that he had only one thought on his mind – to finish in time so as not to be reprimanded. There was a lot of wood left to chop and stack, and winter was fast approaching. If he completed splitting the cord of wood, he would be welcomed to supper. If not, supper would wait, and he would be chopping in the encroaching darkness. Supper would grow cold, but not so cold as the heart of his father, Tom thought. He worked harder and tried to go faster and as he thought about it all, tears ran down his face in frustration. It wasn't just the amount of work, or the difficult tasks set before him by his dad who seemed to be harder on Tom than on his elder brothers, it was the unending bleakness of it all.

There was no joy to be had on the Law farm – never a word of praise nor gratitude or respect from his dad. To add to his frustration, it seemed his mother was almost afraid to show any kind of affection for him unless they were alone. As he chopped and fought to stop the tears streaming down his cheeks, he vowed to himself to never put a family of his own in this kind of situation. There had to be a better life somewhere, and he would find it.

Lost in these bleak thoughts, he was unaware that he had started on the second cord, and his dad yelled out the door to him, "Come on in to supper now, Tom. You can finish the next cord tomorrow night after chores." Tom was eleven years old.

None of the boys were ever close to their dad. The elder Law was not given to any sort of show of emotion and most especially any demonstration of love for his sons. He was typical of some of the men in those days, tough both physically and mentally with little room for any show of affection - even for his wife - and certainly not for the boys. He felt the family was basically there to enhance and further the maintenance of the family coffers and the children, especially boys, were not to be coddled. He attempted to bring them up in the same manner he had been taught by his father before him and felt boys needed to be tough to survive.

Every once in a while, however, Tom would catch a glimpse of compassion from his mother. She had been raised in a town by loving parents, who were unhindered in their ability to nurture and openly show their affection for their children. Her family was financially more stable, so she had received the basics of an education. Because of this, she had a greater inclination toward a balance in life and so she was able to give the boys some of the nurturing that was so sadly lacking otherwise.

Tom was her favorite and the baby of the family. She encouraged him in everything he did, and as a result he spent most of his time with her when his chores were finished. Because of the few moments and stolen energy she allowed for the boys, especially Tom, his fondest childhood memories centered on his mother – memories that were often so simple as sharing a special bowl of soup that she would make for only the two of them.

Sometimes, when Tom's two older brothers were at school, Tom would help his mother carry the washed clothes out to the clothesline. He would try his best to reach the line and help her hang them to dry in the sunshine. Occasionally they would listen to an opera on the radio together – stolen moments – mother and son alone, and an indelible impression was made on Tom of those times spent together.

Unfortunately, the more Tom's mother helped Tom, the more his dad became suspicious of him, and it was expressed in myriad ways. Tom attempted to understand his father's reasoning, but it was incomprehensible. Furthermore, it seemed to Tom that his dad went out of his way to humiliate him, to poke fun at him whenever he could. Some of the situations he forced on Tom seemed to backfire, and while it should have been gratifying, there was little solace.

One such occasion occurred when Tom's dad told everyone in town that Tom was, for all intents and purposes, just basically stupid. Several men had gathered on the porch of the local hardware store owned by Genevieve's parents. Tom's dad felt this was his opportunity to not only profess his own significance, but also make fun of and belittle his son, and to add icing on the cake, get a dig into his in-laws.

"That boy just can't hardly write his name – sure won't amount to anything if I know the likes of him." He nodded to the other men who were standing and leaning against the storefront.

The men snickered and one of them said, "Yeah, well, hey Orley, I heard your boy's been asked to give a speech for one of those clubs next week. Been asked to represent the high school." His smile was friendly, albeit missing a front tooth.

"Shhhzeee, he can't barely read, can't imagine any speech he'd give. All that boy ever does is burn daylight. Gets it from his mother's side," Orley said, and with that, he spit and sauntered off, feeling a deep sense of satisfaction.

It was the next week that a very nervous Tom gave the speech in front of a large group of men at one of the local business organizations. His speech was about American Patriotism, and while Tom had never spoken publicly before, he felt that this was an opportunity to express himself. The grown men listened attentively, and at the end, applauded for a long time. Tom was exultant, and looked into the crowd to find his father's face, but when their eyes met, his father looked away.

At the end, Orley Law walked out without a word to Tom. No congratulations, no praise. Tom didn't really expect more, but it deepened his anger. There would never be any pleasing his father. When he mentioned it to his mother, she just smiled and told Tom that she was very proud, and that he should not expect too much from his father. There were, after all, other things on his father's mind.

As it turned out, Tom was soon to find out what preoccupied his father. Orley had a penchant for being an entrepreneur. He knew instinctively the emerging trends, and while he had never quite caught the tides of change, he had ideas. Some ideas had merit, he thought to himself, but it was always hard to tell. Success was the only measure of a man, and ideas came and went with the seasons. His latest discovery was moonshine. It was illegal to make or to buy; yet there was definitely a demand.

The techniques for making moonshine were zealously guarded, and the stills were considered family heirlooms – passed down from generation to generation. It was a dangerous proposition to attempt to locate a source, as the government sent special agents, called Revenuers, out on a regular basis into the wilderness to find and destroy the stills. As a result, moonshine was hard to come by. People had been shot at who didn't know the proper way to approach a place to buy corn liquor, and since ninety-nine percent of the moonshiners never touched a drop of the corn liquor themselves, they tended to be formidable marksmen.

The whole process of safety and secrecy in buying corn liquor was called, "The Blind Pig" in this area, for reasons that were not certain. What was certain that given the limited supply and the large demand, Mr. Law had the notion that there was a unique business opportunity here, if one could only get past the initial obstacles. Knowing the risks, Orley decided that there should be a fair mark-up of the price, if he could just establish a ready source. It also followed that a small boy would be a harder target to hit, so logic dictated that Tom might stand a better chance of not getting shot than himself.

One Sunday morning, Orley launched his plan. "Get in the car, Tom, we're going for a ride."

"Where?" Tom asked, and then growing suspicious said, "I still have chores to do Dad."

"Never mind the chores, Tom. You've been working hard. Time for a break. You're special, heard you speak in front of everyone, so I want to teach you about business."

Tom, still suspicious asked, "Does mom know about this?"

"No," Orley said, "and if you know what's good for you, she won't. You got that? Not a word to her." Tom's heart sank, and he reluctantly climbed into the truck.

As the old Ford bumped down the country road, Tom ventured a guess as to where they were headed. "Are we after firewood?" he asked.

"Tom," Orley answered, "I'm going to teach you something special today – something very important."

"What?" Tom asked.

"Well, it's part of a business see, a business that we're going into together, just me and you and it'll help our family with some extra money. Maybe you can buy something you want for yourself." Tom looked disdainfully out the window. He knew the family would never see any of whatever money that might be made, but there was very little he could do about it.

"You're going to help me buy moonshine and I'm going to show you just how to do it."

"Moonshine?!" Tom couldn't believe his ears. Even at *his* age he had heard adults talking about how dangerous it was to buy, and how Mr. Vetervo had been shot and his poor, ol' body had been drug away up into the hills.

Some of the kids had said that the moonshiners had thrown his body into a still where it had rotted and turned into moonshine liquor itself.

His brothers had said it was the truth – so help them God. Tom still wasn't sure he believed them, but he did know it was a dangerous thing to do. He looked at his dad and wondered why he would want him to be a part of it.

His dad caught Tom's look and quickly said, "Now, look, Tom. We're going to drive to a road where it's only about umm…a half mile or so from where the moonshiners live – well, at least they live somewhere around there. But," he looked sidelong at Tom who was now slumped deep into the seat with his arms crossed. "But," he said again, "We can't drive up the road you see."

"Why not?" Tom wanted to know.

"Cause, what you have to do is this. We'll park the car off the side of the road in a certain spot and then we get out, turn around very slowly – so they can see us plainly – and then you'll take this quarter and walk very slowly up the road. Somewhere up the path you'll see a, sort of table made out of a board that's set across two other boards that…"

"Why do *I* need to do it?" Tom interjected. Tom knew when he said the words, he shouldn't have. His dad raised his hand as if to strike him, but seemed to think better of it and grabbed the steering wheel again. His dad looked straight ahead at the narrowing road. The road was rutted and bumpy, and Tom's teeth chattered, partly from the bumps and partly from his nerves. The trees and bushes were becoming thicker and started encroaching on the road. Potholes that were filled with rainwater deepened, and the truck bumped and splashed laboriously through them.

The road seemed to go on forever to Tom. In his mind, he pictured that soon he would be lost up in the remote wilderness, and probably, a few days later, his body would be rotting in a still - supplementing the corn liquor just like Mr. Vetervo. He hoped it would at least taste bad and that someone would notice and call the Revenuers.

The truck came to a slow stop, and Orley turned off the motor and sat there for a minute, not saying anything. "You're gonna do this for me, Tom, and that's just it." His dad looked at him and Tom knew it was over on his part. There was no arguing now. "And don't you start your crying either, Tom. It's dangerous enough and if you're making a fuss, you'll only make an easier target." Tom started to fidget, but his dad whispered through his teeth, "Sit still and don't move, not even a finger."

By now Tom was terrified and his chin started to quiver. He hated it when it did that. Hated it because he knew if his dad saw it, he would make fun of him, but right now he noticed his dad seemed to be a little scared too.

After about five minutes of just sitting and breathing, Tom's dad said, "O.K. Now, we're going to get out of the truck slowly and turn around – slowly, a few times. Then I'll give you the quarter so they can see you have it and you'll start walking up the road – very slowly and with your eyes on the ground right in front of you. Don't even think of looking anywhere else, Tom, just look at the road directly in front of you and keep your eyes down.

You understand?"

Tom couldn't even utter a word. He was, by this time, scared speechless. His eyes were as big around as saucers and all he could think about was being home. Home. He knew he'd never see home or his mother again.

"Tom!" His dad hissed through his teeth. "I asked do you understand what you're supposed to do?" His dad mumbled something under his breath and Tom reached for the handle of the truck. His doom was sealed and at the hand of his own father.

Tom opened the door, but his knees were shaking so hard he couldn't make them move until his dad reached over with his hand held low in the seat and pinched Tom on the rear end. It caused him to shoot out of the door much faster than he intended and now, now he knew for sure he'd be killed. Tears sprang to his eyes, but he didn't dare wipe them.

They walked to the front of the truck, stood with their arms out and slowly turned around three times. Then Tom's dad ceremoniously took the quarter out of his pocket and placed it in Tom's outstretched palm, gave him a little shove up the road and leaned back against the hood of the truck.

Tom glanced at his dad and started walking up the side of the road, much too fast and his dad once again hissed through his teeth, "Slower you…and keep your eyes down like I told you!"

Tom obeyed and slowly walked up the dirt road that soon turned into nothing more than a path with deep crevasses. By now, Tom was more than uncomfortable. The forest was too close on both sides – anyone could grab him and pull him into the woods – thus ending his life.

Every shadow seemed alive and filled with moonshiners with guns pointed at his head – just waiting to drag him into the woods and throw his body into a big pot where he would boil away until nothing was left of him but bones – then he'd become moonshine.

He walked slowly at first and then, as any ten year old would do, began to adjust to the whole idea. The road had taken several turns and it had been quite awhile since his dad could see him. He was on his own, but he was used to that.

After a half-mile or so he picked up his pace and almost forgot that he was supposed to walk straight ahead with his eyes down. But maybe there really isn't anyone there, he thought to himself. Maybe this was just an old path that led to a house where they were giving out food – Tom was hungry and that feeling almost took over his being scared.

Suddenly he heard noises in the woods – something like voices yelling and then a loud pop like a gun going off. It jarred him back to reality and his teeth started to chatter.

He kept his eyes directly on the road and walked as slow as he could and as he went around the next curve, there it was.

A long, jagged board was fixed across a three-foot area between two trees. It was cut out on either end to fit the trees, and it made a sort of table. Tom walked up to it and sat his quarter on the board, then slowly backed away as his dad had told him to do. He backed almost all the way down to the curve then turned around and walked slowly on past an area that conveniently put the wooden table out of sight. He waited what seemed to him to be an eternity, then he heard a soft whistle – a sign he could go back to the table.

Turning around, he walked slowly back past the curve and up to the table where, to his relief, there stood a large jug of moonshine.

Tom took the jug and started back down the path to the road, but he forgot that he was to walk slowly and in the same manner that he walked up. He was almost running when suddenly he heard a loud shot ring out and shatter the branch of a tree about six feet ahead of him. Tom froze and waited. He would be dead if he made that mistake again, and cursing at himself for forgetting, he began again – ever so slowly – to walk back to the truck. When he reached it his dad was jubilant.

"What'd I tell you son! That wasn't so hard, was it?"

"They shot at me," Tom said flatly.

"Eh? How's that?" Tom's dad was busy inspecting the contents of the jug. "They shot at you? Thought I heard something. Well, they must have meant to miss, so next time just be more careful."

Tom was disgusted at the lack of concern from his dad, but too drained and relieved to care much about it at the time. At least he had survived, he thought.

Over the next few years Tom made hundreds of "Blind Pig" runs. It eventually became routine, and the fear of dying was replaced by the simple drudgery of routine. It was not without profit, since Tom's dad had been right, there was a demand for the product and the venture was profitable. As a supplement, Orley had found some sources deep in the hills for handmade pottery. Purchasing the crockery for pennies apiece, he was able to re-bottle the moonshine and add to the mark up. He more than tripled the price of hard corn liquor when he sold it, and now with the jugs available as well, he had a thriving business. All he had to do was find a way to have Tom do all of it for him and still make the money – which he soon accomplished.

In those days a family could license a child to drive at the age of fourteen, and so Tom's dad lied about his age and had him get a license when he was barely twelve. It freed Orley's time and Tom, who at first was thrilled with the prospect of driving, soon became disenchanted with the long drives he was forced to make alone. It was obvious all too soon that this was to be one of his jobs and that their "business" together really meant money in his dad's pocket and not a penny in Tom's or anyone else's.

When it came time for Tom to go back to school in the fall, his dad was resistant. The business was being carried by Tom alone, and Orley saw little reason to take away his sole employee. "I'm teaching the boy all he needs to know about business." Orley would say to his wife. "This is our time to be together." But Mrs. Law would not hear of it. Much to Tom's relief, she won the debate, and Tom was allowed to return to his studies. It was not easy, as the other chores still needed attending, and the teachers in the Clarksburg school had little sympathy if a child was required to work until after dark on a homestead. Homework had to be completed, or the marks would be poor.

Consequently, none of the Law boys had much of a chance to excel in school and that was fine with their dad. It meant they would be more likely to stay home and help him on the farm.

But as the school years passed Tom had glimpses into an adult world that he found both puzzling and fascinating at the same time. He was in the 10th grade at Bridgeport High when he was walking home one day with one of his brothers and remembered he had forgotten his homework book

"Better go back and get it, Tom," his older brother Bob said, "You know you have to do the homework – or else."

Their middle brother, Dan had gone home early. Tom ran all the way back to the school only to find everything locked up tight. So he walked around to the back of the school and found an open door.

Once inside, he knew he could get to his class and his homework assignment and books, which were inside his desk. He was walking quietly toward his room when he heard hushed laughing. It sounded like his teacher and someone else, but he couldn't tell whom. Curiosity got the best of him and he peeked around a door just in time to see his teacher, Mrs. Connely, with a man that wasn't her husband - that much he knew as he'd met Mr. Connely several times when he came to pick his wife up and take her home.

They were hugging and kissing, and Tom was so shocked and surprised that he forgot to dart back behind the door. He brushed the door jam and as luck would have it, they both turned toward him and he was caught – and so were they.

Mrs. Connely gasped and said, "Oh, Tom! This isn't what you think…this is my… cousin…" her voice trailed off with the obvious lie… but it was too late anyway, and Tom turned and ran out the door and home.

It was several days before he was able to show up at school again. He left home in the morning and just went down to the river to think. Adults really puzzled him. What makes them do what they do? They always talked about what was right and wrong, but when you caught them with their guard down, they seemed to apply a different set of standards.

Why, Tom wondered, did they say one thing and do another? What motivated people – was it something about the way they thought?

He wanted the answers, but doubted that he would get them from his teachers.

After the episode with his teacher, Mrs. Connely, Tom seemed to lose a lot of his interest in school. As time went on, there were some teachers he liked and tried to please but for the most part, he didn't always show up for a lot of his classes. He had been expelled twice and only by virtue of his mother's insistence did he return.

She pulled him aside one day and sat him down. "Tom," She began, "Why are you ditching school?" Tom looked up at her, and struggled with his conscience. He wanted to tell her that he felt it was a waste of time, echoing his father's words in a moment of convenience, but he knew she would hear nothing of it. Also, he thought, if his father objected so much to an education, then there must be a good reason to have one. This was, he realized, one of the few ways in which he could secretly rebel.

"I'm tired, Mom," he said, finally.

"We all are sweetheart," she said, "But you only have a couple more years to go. You can do it, Tom. I know you can." She was looking at him, and he thought he saw her eyes tearing. It disturbed him more than harsh words ever could have.

"You want to make a life for yourself, don't you, Tom?"

"I'll work harder, Mom, I promise."

"It's not just a matter of hard work, Tom. It's that you have to start using your mind. You have a good one, even though you've never had much of a chance to prove it, but you're smart enough. Find a way to learn, Tom. Learn everything you can, while you have the chance. That's the only way you'll ever get away from here."

His mother's voice trailed off, then she walked away, leaving Tom alone to think.

He considered the schoolwork, and what it was he supposed to be learning, but much of it didn't seem to apply to life. Still, there were things he was curious about, and he determined to apply himself in school for his mother if for no other reason.

One month later, in English, Tom was caught again breaking the rules. He was sitting at his desk reading from the school textbook. He was holding it up in front of him while slouching down in his chair. He became so engrossed that he didn't see Mrs. Carpenter walking by.

Her hand slowly pulled the book down to the desktop, exposing the hidden book Tom had carefully concealed. It was a tattered copy of King Henry the Fourth. Tom had never read Shakespeare before, and his absorption and lack of attention to the classroom around him would now cost him dearly.

Mrs. Carpenter regarded Tom for a moment while he waited for the punishment that was sure to follow, but instead, she smiled a quick smile and then becoming serious said, "Just stick to your school assignment for now, Tom."

He quickly put away King Henry and dove into the reader, grateful for the unexpected amnesty. During the rest of the week, Juanita Carpenter began to pay more attention to Tom. She pulled him aside one day and gave him an extra reading assignment.

"I want you to read this poem by Wordsworth, Tom. Then I want you to tell me what it means to you."

Tom read the poem late that night under the covers of his bed by flashlight. It was beautiful. He read several others before drifting off to sleep, and the next day he met Mrs. Carpenter after class.

"It's about life," Tom said.

She smiled and said, "What about it, Tom? What does it mean here? The part that says, 'Our soul that rises with us, our life's star, hath had elsewhere it's setting, and commeth from afar'?"

"It means," Tom said, "He means that the world is turning, and as one star sets, another rises."

"That's very good. You understand it." She was smiling at him.

"It's not that hard," Tom said, "I read several others too."

"I'm sure you did," Mrs. Carpenter said. "I have a job for you, Tom. I want you to be the Editor of the school newspaper. You can write about all the things that happen around the school, just as long as I get to see what you have written before we print anything."

"How much time will it take?" Tom asked, "I have chores at home...."

"You don't have to write everything, Tom. You'll just have to help. I just want you to read what's written, and if it needs correction or changes, you make suggestions about it."

"OK," Tom said, then he considered, "I can only write about the things that happen here at school?"

Mrs. Carpenter laughed briefly, "No, Tom, you can write about things happening in the world, if you like. But most people around here are going to be more interested in local events."

Tom had another thought then asked, "I can write about individual people here at school, and what they do?"

Mrs. Carpenter paused, then said, "You may want to be careful with that one, Tom. People like their privacy. There are lots of things you and I may be aware of, but I would never make them known. Try to stick to things that are positive – it will keep you out of a lot of trouble."

Tom understood. It would have been tempting to write an expose on the hypocrisy of adults, but he knew better than that. He accepted his new position with enthusiasm and soon discovered a dormant talent he had in writing.

His year as the Editor was exciting, and the self-esteem he gained as a result gave him the incentive to apply himself to the other courses. By the end of his third year, his improvements in school were significant enough that the faculty awarded him "Boy's State," which was given only once a year to the best student. From near expulsion to significant recognition in school, Tom had proven himself, at least to his mother.

Tom had reservations, however, as his overall memory of academics was of a brief moment of glory, buried beneath many years of failure. For the most part, Tom shared his father's viewpoint that he was not particularly bright.

It was the next July after graduation that Tom turned eighteen and the Second World War was in full swing. Tom didn't have any idea what he was going to do with his life so when the Sea Bees drafted him, it was a relief. Several of his school friends that lived on farms were drafted into the Sea Bees too, as they already knew how to run tractors and heavy equipment and were considered valuable commodities by virtue of their experience.

Tom found it easy to leave his family, even going into the unknown of the military. His father, in an ironic way, had prepared him for hardships.

He was willing to go anywhere and do anything as long as it was away from the belittling condescension of his dad. The only reluctance he felt was in leaving his mother.

From the poem Homestead…

First they built the barn. Come winter storm.
In those staggered hills, the cold would kill a cow.
Some nights the avalanche of crystal wind tumbling down the coal-cold
slopes
Would shiver the harp strings of the taut-strung pines; left just one night
in the open
It would lock the animals in ice - like mammoths.
Before the kids and woman, they kept the livestock warm.
It snowed a lot on that Blue Ridge. Nobody was ever quite warm, nobody
ever really got dry.
Slowly the babies came, the loft filled; two years or so there was another,
and the need for wool to spin a blanket, milk for older kids snatched
early from the breast, wood lye and lard for soap, hog and harvest for
them all.

It was a big house.
Thirteen rooms with fireplaces for each.
Nine rooms for the children,
One room for the pair that launched the babies
On the gaunt trajectory from pillow to plow.
Two warm rooms saved to welcome friends and kin
Uncommon come on holy days from yon side of the hills
To share the abundance of the fields, furrow, marriage bed.
It was how they endured.

They're all dead now.
Those hard, strong men, those enduring women:
How could they die, how could they ever die?
Mother said,
"They worked themselves to death."

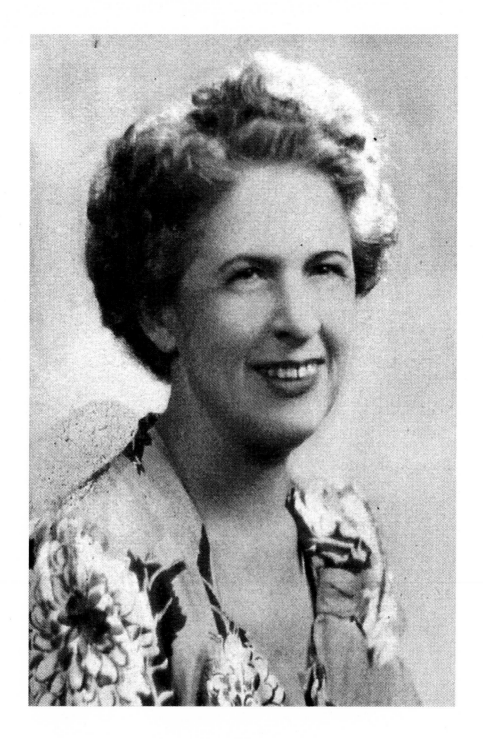

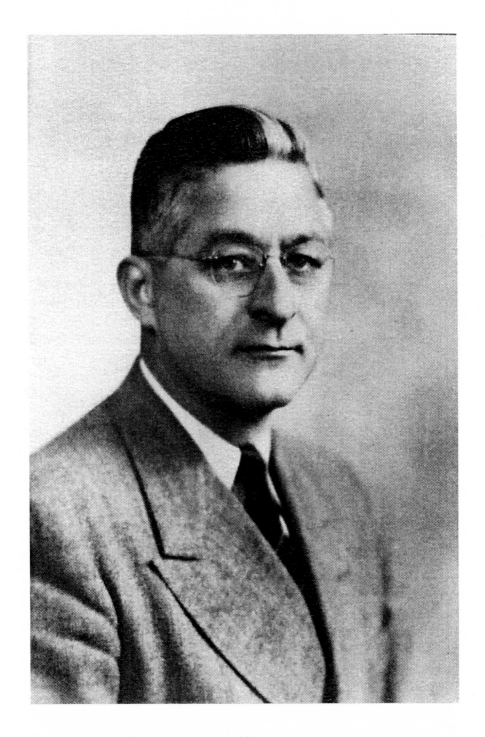

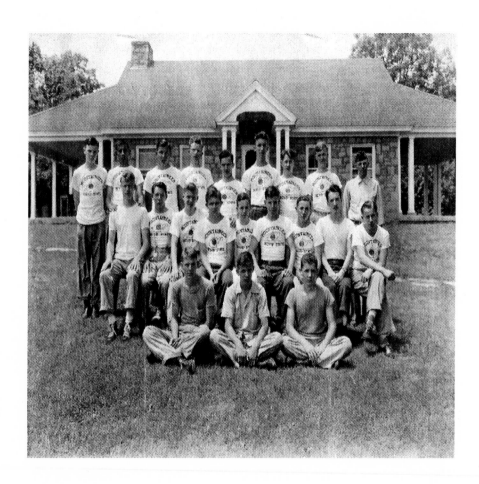

Chapter Three

A voice behind, grim with the habit of authority, spoke in an indictment of offense…

Mike smiled at Tom and gave a "thumbs up" sign right before the loader he was running placed the final box on the top of the pile of other crates. It was his last act and it sealed Tom into his own, very private world. The forklift made a grinding sound as Mike backed up and went on rearranging the loaded crates that sat on pallets in the immense warehouse. The Navy's Construction Battalion, aka Sea Bee's, had its own way of doing things and this storage building was living proof. Tons of items from toilet paper to toothbrushes, as well as typewriters, desks, even food supplies comprised the inner workings of the support system for the Navy. All of it needed to be accounted for, yet there were so many steps involved that no private industry could have operated in this manner.

There was a constant shuffle of items coming and going with the purpose of supplying all the men stationed at this base in Honolulu. The record of those items was endless and by its very nature, constantly changing.

This was the 101st Construction Battalion situated on the Moana Loa Ridge. The 101st was later to become the Advanced Base Construction Depot. They were responsible for both building and shipping construction materials all over the world during the 2nd World War.

The warehouse itself sat on several acres and became the main supply depot or exchange storage for the Sea Bee's since the beginning of World War II. From here, items as large as bulldozers and backhoes were shipped anywhere and everywhere when they were needed around the world.

Mike was only one of any number of men that worked the warehouse with task lists as long as their arms. Because of the vast amount of items, usually one man took care of an assigned section. He was the one in charge of moving the thousands of crates and keeping track of the inventory.

Mike first met Tom while standing in the chow line one morning. He had seen him around, but there were always new men in the Sea Bee's. They had a continual rotation of men both arriving and shipping out. Mike happened to line up right behind Tom one day, and to his amazement, watched him read an instructional book on the Japanese language.

"What's reading that book about?" he asked Tom with a smile.

"Oh, just learning the language – or at least trying to."

Tom was just about to say he thought he might be of some help to his government when he looked up to see the Master at Arms approaching from behind, checking each man as he passed by. As he reached Tom and Mike he looked at the book Tom held in his hand. The title of the book was in bold, and said, "Learning Japanese."

"Hey sailor, you don't read in *my* chow line. What kind of Japcrap are you reading anyway?" He yanked the book out of Tom's hand and started yelling at the top of his lungs. Both Tom and Mike were taken back as the Chief exploded - the blood veins in his neck were protruding. "We're at W-A-R in case you hadn't noticed sailor and it happens to be *with* the Japs, fer Christ's sake!" The veins in his neck were pulsing, and bulged all the further.

Mike and Tom stood at attention and said, "Yes! Chief!"

The Chief started ripping the book apart page-by-page and dropping it on the ground where it was blown across the compound by the trade winds that were in full force that morning.

"You can pick every piece of this paper up, Law, and you can help, Stoddard! Don't ever let me catch you reading in chow line again and *never* a book about our enemies – do I make myself *very* clear?"

"Yes Chief!"

"Whew," Mike said rolling his eyes, who was still stunned by the overreaction of the Chief, "I can't believe that, can you?"

Tom shook his head, and while he and Mike scrambled to pick up as many of the fragments of the book as they could, he said, "Sorry, Mike. You had nothing to do with this – sorry you were pulled into it."

"Yeah," Mike said, "I think I could have told you that reading in chow line was a stupid thing to do. But don't worry, most of the book is blown off base now anyway. We still have time to get back in line."

Tom looked back to the line. It was getting shorter. They could slip in at the end and still have something to eat.

"I don't get it though, Law, why a book on Japanese? I mean, a skin magazine I could understand, but *Japanese*?" Mike said.

Tom dumped his wad of papers into a bin, and taking Mike's handful, threw the last of them in the trash. "Believe it or not, Stoddard, I think I can help our cause. For some reason I find language easy to learn, and besides, why *wouldn't* we want to know the language of our enemies? What if we are captured? What if we intercept a transmission? Wouldn't it be a *good* thing to be able to translate it?"

Mike snorted, and then said, "In case you hadn't noticed Law, you're enlisted. You're for washing dishes and moving boxes. You're a grunt. They have the brains from the Academies working on that other stuff."

"I know, I know," Tom said, "But a month ago I snuck into a class on base – a language class. I understand it. I can learn it, and even though I'm just an enlisted, some of these things are easy for me. Now, I don't know what to do. The instructor thinks I'm in his class and I can't study. I'll either have to drop it or find some other way – some place where Master Chief can't bust me."

Back at the end of chow line now, they eagerly accepted the plops of nutritious, yet unrecognizable servings onto their trays without comment.

They sat down and Mike gave Tom a slap on the back.

"Don't worry ol' buddy, I have an idea about your study space. If you insist on saving us from the Japs, the least I can do is give you the chance. I'll build you your own office where no one will ever find you. You can study all you want. Although," Mike said musing, "I don't know how you've managed to pull off a class at the base university."

"I just walked in," Tom said between bites, and then when the rest of Mike's comments hit him he said, "What do you *mean*, my own space?"

Tom was skeptical, but it was a nice gesture from a person that he had only met a few minutes before.

"Leave that to me," Mike said, "Just give me a few days and I'll get back to you on it."

Tom smiled and finished eating. He looked up in dismay as a stray paper with Japanese lettering blew across the table, but no one was looking and he and Mike pretended not to notice.

It was barely two days later when Mike rushed up to Tom as he headed for the morning chow line again.

"Wait up, Law. I have good news for you." Mike looked around to make sure no one was listening.

Tom turned around and looked in all directions too, nervous from the other morning when they both had their asses chewed by the Master at Arms.

Tom smiled, "What, Stoddard?"

Stoddard hesitated, and then said, "Remember I promised you something?

Well, I'm a guy you can depend on. I come through for my friends."

"OK," Tom said, as he started walking again towards the line, "So, I am guessing that you talked to the commander, and he agreed to let me have some of his office space so I can study, am I right?"

Mike looked hurt. "You're so right," he said, and then continued, "No. Seriously, I need you to come by the warehouse this afternoon. You'll find me in the back section, OK?"

"Sure," Tom said, "I'll stop by."

When Tom quietly slipped into the back of the enormous warehouse that afternoon, Mike was loading and moving crates in all directions. The loader was large and noisy and Tom had to get in front of him and wave his arms to get his attention. Mike smiled and hopped off the loader, but left it running, motioning Tom to follow him.

He had arranged an 'office' complete with desk and chair behind several heavy crates that were piled almost to the ceiling on four sides except for a small vertical opening. The 'door' was positioned toward the back of the boxed-in office and almost up against the back wall of the warehouse itself. Mike had protruded the crates used for the wall out from the other side of the door so the opening was barely noticeable. Actually, if you were standing in the walkway where you could move, you wouldn't notice anything unusual at all. It would take a special effort to find the hidden doorway.

Mike had done some thinking about all this beforehand. He used only crates that were not due to leave or even be moved for quite a while, and then he arranged them so the dates were clearly visible. The ones most likely to be shipped first were the ones on the top. For all intents and purposes, Tom's stolen office was as permanent and secure as any other on the base.

"You did all *this*?" Tom said with a mixture of gratitude and disbelief.

"Check it out," Mike said, "It's small but hidden. The only catch is that you won't be able to get out until I move the crate out of the way, but we can arrange a schedule. Just let me know how long you plan to be in there, and I'll be back to open it up for you."

"I don't believe it, Mike," Tom said, "Thanks."

Mike smiled and ushered Tom into the office, and with a flourish, he showed him the desk and small lamp. It was perfect. Tom ran back to his barracks and returned with a bag full of books. He told Mike to bring him out in four hours and gave a "thumbs up" as Mike lifted a heavy crate on the forklift and sealed Tom into his private world.

Four hours later, Mike returned to the back of the warehouse and opened the hidden space. Tom was hunched over his books, having hardly moved from the moment that Mike left him.

"Time's up," Mike said, "Same time tomorrow?"

"Same time," Tom said, "and Mike, thanks again. This is going to be great."

Mike replaced the crate after Tom left and closed the warehouse for the night.

"Japanese," he muttered and thought to himself; personally, I would have taken about a hundred different courses before that. He shrugged to himself and walked off.

Tom used his private warehouse office consistently over the next few months and studied Japanese, along with several other courses. Cryptography was interesting, and there were other books that he had chanced upon and borrowed. If he combined a working knowledge of several languages, he might stand a chance at deciphering. It was a long shot, he admitted to himself, that anyone would allow him the opportunity, but his instructor at the university had already said that Tom was near the top of the class, and with a little leverage, he might make a new grade. It was breaking the rules, but that wasn't troublesome to Tom. He felt rules existed for that singular purpose. Besides, he thought, his regular duties were only about half of what he had been required to do as a child on the farm. What others complained about as backbreaking labor, Tom found to be a partial workload. He had time and energy left over at the end of the day and boredom drove him to find more activity.

Tom studied continuously. He applied his mind to philosophy, language and carefully examined several other disciplines. He nearly memorized "The Communist Manifesto" by Karl Marx. That was a dangerous endeavor, he realized, but safe within his fortress, he could let his mind explore. It was fascinating, all of it. Karl Marx had a good point, Tom thought, although Marx was naïve to think that people would work for a "common good." It was a noble thought, but inherently flawed. People worked because they had to. Nothing more. Life in Appalachia had taught him that much at an early age. He felt that Marx had probably led a coddled, idealistic life. The luxury of having too few things to do on any given day.

Tom's Japanese was progressing nicely, and he began to work on simple cryptographic codes. It would not be long before he could approach his commanding officer and surprise him with a certificate of completion in language.

Unfortunately, Tom was in for a disappointment. Several of the other enlisted men had noticed Tom's habits, and they felt that Tom stayed aloof out of a feeling of superiority. Tom rarely went out with the other enlisteds, and when he did, he made the mistake of opening his mouth and sounding intelligent.

One of the men followed Tom one day to the warehouse out of curiosity and reported to the Chief Storekeeper that there was a violation. The next day, the Chief followed Tom at a safe distance, so as not to be detected, and discovered the clandestine operation.

The Chief waited until Mike had placed the last crate, and then said in a loud voice, "OK, Stoddard, Where's Law!"

Mike froze in place, and then before he could answer, Tom yelled from inside the enclosure, "In here, sir!"

Tom didn't want Mike to get into any more trouble than he no doubt already was, so after Mike started the loader and moved the boxes, Tom walked out of his private office for the last time. The Chief Storekeeper marched them both down to the Lieutenant in charge where they were interviewed separately and then together.

Tom said the whole thing had been his idea – that he was trying to learn the Japanese language in order to be of service to his country and he couldn't find a place quiet enough to study. Satisfied they were both telling the truth and recognizing the advantage Tom would be able to give to the proper departments, the officers relaxed.

They called a representative from the language department where Tom had taken advanced Japanese and verified that the instructor knew him. They also verified that Tom had taken the course without authorization, but the instructor vouched for Tom, saying that he was one of the best students he had ever taught. The Navy Language School, it seemed, was impressed enough with Tom's proficiency to qualify him in Japanese and to send him to the front as a Military Government Interpreter.

Two weeks later, Tom received his orders to leave for Okinawa. He was to advance with the Marine Corps into the mountains where the Japanese soldiers were in hiding. His job would be to explore the caves in the mountains that housed the Japanese and try to convince the soldiers to surrender. It was a position that held little hope for survival, but there were few Americans that had proficiency enough to attempt communication. If unsuccessful, Tom was assured, the remains of the interpreter would be highly honored back in the United States.

Tom was prepared to go, but wondered to himself about his fate in life. His mother had successfully convinced him that knowledge was freedom, yet this was actually far *worse* than being shot at by moonshiners. Most of the indigents in Appalachia had muzzle-loading, black powder rifles, and while they were deadly accurate, at least it took them some time to reload. A cave filled with paranoid Japanese soldiers, probably possessing modern rifles, was a big step in the wrong direction.

Tom waited for his shipping out orders and kept in communication with Stoddard. Mike, he found, had gotten off with a minor reprimand. It seemed that the Navy was, by and large, grateful to have a new interpreter, so they let Mike go with a slap on the hand.

Days passed slowly while Tom waited to leave. He decided to spend some of his extra time in social activity, and since he could not read alone undisturbed or attend classes, he began to frequent the bars at night.

One evening he met a Japanese girl. She had somehow avoided relocation into a camp, possibly through political connections. Tom was lonely, and the girl was attractive, so Tom bolstered his courage and asked her out on a date. She was curious about him and the motives he carried. He explained enough about his past assignment in the Sea Bees to satisfy her, all the while steering clear of his current assignment which was highly classified. After some discussion, she acquiesced.

His new girlfriend became friendly, and one evening she invited Tom over to her home. When they were inside the tiny apartment that was little more than one room in the basement of a large home, she asked Tom to sit and be comfortable, while she changed her clothes. Tom waited expectantly. This girl was the finest thing he had met in months, and he wanted desperately to impress her.

She returned from her tiny bedroom dressed in a beautiful, flowing gown just as the phone rang. Smiling at Tom, she answered it, and then asked him to excuse her for a moment until she had finished her call. She left the room, but Tom was able to overhear the conversation. It was in Japanese and seemed to be centered on a cousin that was diabetic and suffering in a concentration camp.

Tom waited politely for the conversation to end. He had not meant to eavesdrop, but at the same time, he wanted to impress this beautiful girl, so when she returned to the room he asked her, in Japanese, how her cousin was getting along.

A look of complete astonishment came over the girl's face and her entire demeanor quickly changed.

"Who are you?" she snapped, as she dropped the phone back onto the cradle. Obviously, he immediately became a suspect of some sinister plot. "Why are you here?" she demanded. Before Tom could answer, she said, "Out. You are leaving right now."

"So I speak Japanese..." Tom started, but she cut him off.

"Out. You set me up, get away." And she shoved him out the door. Tom allowed himself to be pushed outside, then turned away and walked back to base.

Once again, he said to himself, I cut my own throat. Once again, I put my foot in it and opened my mouth. Tom walked away saddened. It was not just that he was a misfit – he had grown used to that. It was just that here was a pretty girl, and if he had kept his thoughts to himself, he would be having a much better time than walking alone back to the barracks. After a few minutes he thought to himself, at least I know one thing for certain; my Japanese is pretty good.

One week later Tom and his platoon were set to ship out. They were packed, and all their gear was stowed in preparation for departure. It was a beautiful morning in Oahu and as the sun rose over the volcano, their thoughts were of the stark contrast this serenity would have with the violence that lay ahead. Here, the sun was just coming up over the horizon, the trade winds had started moving gently up the volcanic mountains toward the top where, in the afternoon they'd gently rush back down the mountain to the sea as they had for thousands of years. Yet what lay ahead was death and despair. Even if the climate might be similar, the situation held little promise for an appreciation of natural beauties.

The men were nervous. It had been a long wait, and the anticipation was grueling. Better, they thought, to get on with it. Leave for their mission and if they survived, get it over with and go home.

Prepped and heading for chow, they were startled by an announcement on the PA system. The thought of another attack by the enemy was always looming constantly in the background, so the announcement took them totally by surprise.

The loud speaker crackled, and they froze in place anticipating the worst.

They waited, and the voice of their Commander came across.

He cleared his voice and said, "Attention all personnel …I have good news this morning. I just received word from Headquarters announcing that the war is officially over! All ships are returning to Home Port. Belay all orders for departure." The Commander paused, then continued, "This day will be remembered by all of us for the rest of our lives." The commander's voice choked with emotion and joy, and he abruptly ended his message.

Tom stood amidst a crowd of jubilant sailors – hats were thrown into the air and chaos broke loose. Tom said a silent prayer of thanks to providence and bumped through the crowd to the officers club, which was opened to everyone in celebration. There, he found Stoddard and they toasted together the fact that it was over, and they had never even seen action.

"To the Sea Bee's," Mike said.

"To farm equipment and fork lifts," Tom said, and they clinked their glasses.

Tom arrived in San Francisco four days later. There was a plane ticket waiting for him at the airline counter. It was a one-way ticket with the ultimate destination of West Virginia, the latter part paid for by his mother. Tom knew he would be excited to see her, but wondered about the reception he would receive. His mother would be emotional, and his father would ask too many questions. Still, he thought, it would be good to go home.

Chapter Four

Freedom With Responsibility
(The Law Family Creed)

Mike and Tom stood outside the bus station in Boston and set their heavy duffle bags on the wet sidewalk. They were still in uniform and hadn't slept for nearly twenty-four hours. Mike had family in New York, and Tom was headed for West Virginia, but neither of them were in a hurry to go home. They might have been, except for the fact that everywhere they went they received a hero's welcome, and the praise and adulation was distracting. A taxi was unnecessary; the Navy uniform was all that was required to get a ride to go anywhere they wanted. Restaurant waiters ushered them to the best seats, and movie theaters often gave them free admission. Back home, they realized, their families waited, but there they would be known for themselves – welcomed and embraced, but hardly war heroes. At any rate, they had to go through military discharge and were stuck in Boston for at least a couple of weeks.

"What do you want to do?" Mike asked. "Find some girls?" he added hopefully.

"Absolutely," Tom replied, "But let's find our way around first."

They found a map of the city at the bus station and located the USO. Another sailor on the flight to Boston had told them of the free entertainment and the abundance of pretty girls, who, he said with a wink, were anxious to please the men returning from the war.

"A couple of weeks," Mike said, "Not nearly enough time to fit it all in."

They were studying the map while standing on the curb, when a young woman with two children pulled up and offered them a lift.

Tom and Mike climbed in, and she smiled and said, "Where to?"

Her young boys, about the ages of six and eight, stared wide-eyed at Mike and Tom.

"Did you have to kill anyone?" the older boy ventured.

48

"Shush!" his mother said, "That's not polite."

Tom smiled. "That's OK," he said to the mother, then to the boy, "No. Actually neither one of us did."

The boy looked disappointed, so Mike added, "But Tom here was just about to go to the caves in Japan and crawl back into the dark, probably over snakes, and get any Japanese soldiers that were hiding inside."

The boy's eyes lit up. "Really?!"

Tom looked at Mike and grunted, then turned to the mother and said, "We just arrived and have some time here, do you have any suggestions?"

"That depends on what you like, I suppose, but for me, it would be the opera. There's a show tonight, and I think you can get in free if you're in uniform."

Mike was sitting in the back with the two boys, engaged in colorful war stories that grew more fanciful by the minute. He looked up and frowned. "Opera?" he said.

"If it's not out of your way," Tom said, before Mike could object any further, "But we should stow our bags first."

The woman smiled and waited as Mike and Tom got out of the car, ran back into the bus station and found lockers for their bags.

Returning to the street they found her still waiting, so they climbed in and accepted the ride to the opera house. She dropped them cheerily on the curb and drove off.

"Wonder where her husband is?" Mike asked.

"Me too," Tom said, "But I didn't want to bring it up unless she did."

The opera house was an ancient building, with gothic architecture and elaborate buttresses. The show would not be starting for a half hour, but Tom wanted to go in early and look around. After they were given free passes, they made their way in, and Mike complained about the selection of activity for the evening.

"Should have been the USO," he said, "This is a bunch of old people here, not likely to meet anyone interesting at all."

Tom ignored him and made his way to his seat with Mike following behind.

The opera started, and both Tom and Mike sat silent. It was their first exposure to this kind of music, and Tom, at least, found it surpassed anything he had ever experienced. After it was over they left and agreed to return in a couple of nights.

Walking to their quarters from the bus station, Mike asked Tom what he was planning to do when he got home. Tom hadn't wanted to think about it. The ethereal music of the opera still filled his head, and it was a sudden jolt to be pulled back to West Virginia.

"I don't know, Mike," he said, "I don't really have any plans right now. What about you?"

"Well," Mike said, "It's back to New York and my family, for sure. Dad's a pharmacist and owns his own building in downtown Manhattan. He wants me to go to school and take over the family business."

"Are you going to?" Tom asked, curious.

"I guess, eventually," Mike said, "But right now I'm ready for some adventure."

Mike suggested they take a trip away from Boston to explore, but Tom wasn't ready to leave just yet. The experience at the Opera haunted him, and he had been absolutely mesmerized by the sound and beauty of the music. His heart opened, and he immersed himself and reveled in the beauty of the splendid sounds. Enticed now with the culture of the cities, Tom became infatuated. It wasn't long before he found the Boston Symphony, and again listened in rapture. He found the theatrical plays to be consummately impressive, and he snatched every free ticket available. Mike would join him on occasion, but more often Tom went alone. He soon learned that his uniform was considered formal attire and that alleviated the need to buy more clothes.

Tom relished in the Arts, although he had never been exposed to them before. He had never heard an Opera or the Boston Symphony, but he found he couldn't stop going. It was a question his friends asked of him often. "Why," they would say, "the sudden obsession with ancient, outdated music?" Tom couldn't explain it, he viewed it all with an elevated feeling of pleasure and wondered about that very feeling inside him - where did it come from and why, among all of his friends, was he was the only one to experience it?

A whole range of questions about human behavior was beginning to interest Tom, but he didn't understand why. He contemplated and struggled on and off to find the significance in his life. On a long walk one day, when Mike had gone his separate way, Tom wandered into the Harvard University library. Even though he was not a student, his uniform provided admission, and Tom perused the endless rows of books. What would it be like, he wondered, to attend a university like Harvard? He doubted he had the capacity, but the vast amount of knowledge stored here, ready for the taking, was magnetic. Tom left the campus after several hours, and again thought about his future plans. He wondered about Mike's plans. Mike had been a photographer in the Navy Sea Bee's in addition to his duties at the warehouse, and photography had always been Mike's passion. Mike was a realist, though, so photography would probably be abandoned, and he would honor his families' wishes to become a pharmacist.

Tom, on the other hand, had no desire to settle down in West Virginia and help his brothers with the new, family hardware store. Virtually anything looked better than that possibility to him. He tried to block it from his mind and to focus on other things, but he knew that he would have to make some choices in his future – he was just uncertain what they should be.

After several days, Tom and Mike prepared to leave Boston. It was more or less a welcome change for Mike, but Tom dreaded it. He would head home and brace himself for the emotional impact that was sure to disrupt his feelings of serenity and joy that had become a part of this time in a center of cultural enlightenment.

"I'm not ready to go back," Tom confided with Mike, "I hated it on the farm, and I doubt I'll like it any more at the hardware store. I'm glad the war's over, but I'm just not ready to return."

Mike listened attentively. His father would be pressuring him to get started at college and then on to pharmacy school. He felt that it was not such a bad thing, but it seemed like something that could wait.

"I have an idea," he said to Tom, "Why not take a trek somewhere – a long journey, into the wilderness – some place that we can be away, and where your family won't bother you?"

Tom wasn't hard to convince at this point.

"Maybe a trip up the Appalachian Trail?" Tom suggested.

"Now, that sounds great!" Mike responded, "I'll get the gear together and check with you in three weeks, after you've had time to say hello to your family."

"How long a trip do you plan on taking?" Tom asked.

"I don't know – maybe a month – let's just go and see how if feels. We can always go back home when we get tired," Mike said.

Tom said his farewells to Boston, and then made his way for West Virginia. When he arrived, his mother ran out to greet him and squeezed him until he could hardly breathe.

His father was uncommonly friendly and Tom spent several days at home, talking about his experiences and the details of the war. He was growing restless, however, by the time Mike called him from a nearby town.

"You ready?" Mike said. Tom gave Mike directions to his house, and Mike found his way there. After introductions were made, and Tom's family realized they had no choice in the matter, the two prepared for the following day's journey.

"Your family OK with you taking some time off?" Tom asked Mike.

"Nope," Mike said, "They didn't want me to come here at all. But I told them that I suffered from 'post-traumatic syndrome' or something to that effect, and they didn't push the issue."

Tom laughed. "I'm surprised you even know what that is," he said.

"I don't," Mike answered, as he spit out a golden piece of hay he had been chewing on, "I think I heard of it somewhere, and it sounded serious enough to use."

"Well as long as it worked," Tom said smiling. He was excited to go and explore the reaches of Appalachia without the onus of moonshine or obligations.

The Appalachian Trail is a continuously marked footpath that goes from Katahdin in Maine to Springer Mountain in Georgia covering approximately 2,160 miles. The trail is generally traced back to a 1921 article by Benton MacKaye and is known to pass through, in portion, 14 states.

In West Virginia there are barely 2 miles of trail. It crosses the Shenandoah River and continues on into Virginia. Tom and Mike took some of their light gear left over from the service and began their adventure. Front Royal was to be their starting point, and they hitched a ride to a bend in the road that marked the trailhead.

After thanking the driver, an older gentleman who upon seeing the military packs, launched into an endless discussion on his experiences in the First World War, they got out and shouldered their gear and supplies. They brought a tarp, but no tents as there were various shelters placed along the Appalachian Trail.

After a four-hour hike, they came to the first shelter and found it unoccupied. It was a three-sided stone cabin, complete with wooden bunk beds and a water supply.

Moss grew on the north side and hung down in loose strands covering some of the branches of the trees. They had replenished their canteens two miles back at a fresh spring, but the water at the cabin was a welcome site. It was hot and humid, and this would give them the opportunity to rinse off.

The late afternoon sun filtered at an angle through the dogwoods, and Mike took advantage of the lighting to shoot several photos.

"Made it," Tom said with a heavy sigh as he dropped his pack.

Mike finished with his camera and started setting up camp. They had an abundant food supply, since they anticipated staying for several weeks. Tom rummaged through for the first official meal on the trail. The evening passed, and Tom fell asleep early. He spent some time, in his last few minutes awake, thinking about his life. He wasn't ready to go back, and he was not sure when, or even if, he ever would be. Mike, he knew, would want to return after this brief adventure, but Tom thought he could stay out here forever.

After several days on the trail, Mike and Tom found an offshoot. Tom was eager to explore it, but Mike thought it looked like a dead end.

"Let's just keep going, Tom," Mike said, "There are some old mining settlements along this trail, and sometimes there are old miners in them – who are very protective and paranoid, I hear."

Tom snorted, "The last thing you need to worry about is miners," he said, "and besides, by the time I was ten I was trading with moonshiners, who are a *lot* more paranoid."

"All the more reason to leave it alone," Mike argued.

Tom acquiesced but made a mental note. He would come back this way, and maybe take the side journey to see where the small trail ended in the hills.

They continued on the trail, once in awhile meeting a few hikers along the way. Most of them were friendly enough, but they usually had come this way for reasons similar to Tom and Mike. They were dropping out, or away, from civilization. It was a time for many people to re-evaluate life and to adjust to the recent changes brought about by the war.

After two months and many long miles on the trail, Tom and Mike made their way back to civilization. Mike was ready to return; he had his family waiting, but Tom had reservations.

They parted company at a bus station, promising to stay in close contact forever, and Mike bought a ticket to Boston. Tom watched him go, and then hoisted his pack again and turned back the way he came.

Within two hours he was back to the trailhead and working his way North, retracing the steps he and Mike had first taken. By nightfall, he was camped again in the original hut, curled snugly in his bag and watching the stars through the holes in the boards that provided a roof of sorts.

Mike received a letter from Tom two months later. It was postmarked from Front Royal, the closest city to the Appalachian trailhead where they had started their trip.

It said, "I found a place to live in the hills. It's perfect here. I'm not going home. Come out and visit when you get a chance." There was a map drawn on the back of the note, and Mike followed the lines along the trail with his eyes to a point where an "X" marked the "house."

Mike frowned as he reread the letter. It sounded to him like Tom was planning to spend the rest of his natural life in the wilderness, and the thought was disturbing to him. Tom had shown plenty of signs about not wanting to return home, but there was no reason to go to this extreme, Mike thought. He decided to take a trip and search out his friend on his next break from work. He had been working at the pharmacy, waiting until he would begin college at the University of Wisconsin in Madison. After some negotiations with his father, he was able to arrange time off.

"What are you doing, Tom?" Mike asked as he stood there shaking his head in disbelief.

Tom was standing at the opening of a raised corn-crib cabin.

"Welcome traveler!" Tom said, "Welcome to Walden River!"

"What stinks?" Mike asked.

"The river," Tom said, "It has a high sulfur content – probably from some strip-mining upstream. Actually, it's quite medicinal. Cures warts."

"Ugh," Mike said, and then, "I'll remember to take some back with me to the pharmacy. Dad will love it, I'm just sure. And," he added, "could you possibly have gotten any further out into these woods?" Tom climbed down the rickety stairs and helped Mike unload some groceries.

"I chanced on this place by accident," Tom said, "I guess it must have been a farm once. There are about forty acres that were cleared years ago, but a mining company must have come in and taken it over." Mike stopped to inspect his surroundings; it was actually serene and starkly beautiful. Nothing grew by the creek, but there was a water pump that filled a stone cistern. The corn-crib cabin was raised about eight feet off the ground, and inside Tom had arranged a cot and shelves where he had placed a kerosene lantern and several books. It was homey, in a rustic way.

"That road coming out here is really something, Tom. You'd never get out of here if it were raining more than a drop. I've never seen such ruts."

Mike began arranging some groceries he brought in a corner while Tom climbed back down the ladder to help bring up the rest of them.

"I know," Tom said over his shoulder, "But isn't it something? No one comes out here – just the deer and rabbits, and the steps keep them out of the food." Tom rummaged around in Mike's car and came across a pile of books. "What's this?" he asked, "for me?"

Mike joined him and picked up the top book; it was a battered copy of the works of Shakespeare. "You hinted rather heavily that you were in need," Mike said, "So I went to a bookstore in Clarksburg, grabbed everything I could carry."

In the rest of the stack there were volumes of poetry, as well as several novels and a textbook on psychology.

"You're the best," Tom said, and they finished unloading and arranging in the cabin.

Mike straightened up, and with his hands on his hips, looked out at the view from the open front of Tom's borrowed home.

"So, what's the story, Tom? You're planning on living here now? I mean, it's beautiful, don't get me wrong, but just how long do you plan on being out here?"

Tom joined him at the opening. "I don't know, Mike. I really like it. It's high and mostly dry, when it isn't raining, and the price is right. All I need is a lady friend once in awhile and plenty of books to read. What more could I want?"

Mike snorted, "Well good luck finding companionship out here."

"I'm figuring I'll have to import," Tom said.

"I see," Mike said with sarcasm, "No doubt you'll find someone in town who will happily walk the miles out this way."

Tom smiled and started climbing down, "Follow me, I have something to show you." Mike followed Tom to the back of the cabin. There was a tarp covering a bulking object. Tom pulled the tarp off with a flourish, exposing a Harley Davidson motorcycle. It was covered with mud and rust, but intact.

"It runs?" Mike asked.

"All the way into town and back," Tom said beaming, "The perfect chariot, this is, and suitable for bringing in books, supplies and adventuresome souls."

Mike spent several days in the wilderness with Tom, hiking and exploring the vast, lonely area. He had tried to press Tom into making some plans for his future or at the least to look into another line of work besides being a hermit, but Tom wouldn't budge on the issue. "I'm happy here," Tom would say with finality.

Giving it up as a lost cause, Mike agreed to visit on occasion and bring in more books and supplies. After several days, Tom waved goodbye to his friend as the car struggled down the rutted path, and he went back inside.

It was time, he thought, to write some poetry. He missed Mike and started to wonder if he should consider bringing someone else out to the corncrib hermitage.

It was a passing thought that lasted only a moment, and he soon returned to the pen and paper he was balancing on his crossed legs. "Ode to Appalachia" was scrawled on the top line.

A storm moved in across the mountains and dropped buckets of rain. It smelled fresh and settled the dust and even temporally cleaned the river. After a few days though, Tom began to wonder if the rain would ever stop. In resignation, he decided to make the best of it and took the opportunity to read several of the books Mike had brought him, as well as work on some poetry.

One week later, when the rain started to let up, Tom fired up the Harley and headed for Clarksburg. He needed to check in with his family, and he braced himself for their worried comments about his disreputable life.

On the first day he was home, amidst a load of laundry that his mother was fussing over, Tom listened as she begged him to return. He felt bad for her, so to spare her feelings he did not mention that he had no intention of ever returning.

His father was at the hardware store, and Tom elected to avoid him. Tom's older brother, Dan, was home and he watched smiling as their mother completed a load of Tom's wash.

When Dan had a minute alone with Tom, he asked him if he would like to meet some of his friends. Tom agreed, Dan had a reputation of being friendly with the ladies, and Tom knew that his odds of success in meeting someone just increased ten-fold. Tom followed Dan's model A Ford to a park in the center of town, and Dan introduced Tom to several young people gathered there. A picnic table was covered with fried chicken and homemade side dishes. There was a large jar of pickles, and Tom helped himself to one. Between bites, Tom conversed with Dan, who was fascinated by the corncrib cabin Tom had discovered.

"I have to see it!" Dan said, "I can't believe you could be happy out there all alone, so it must be one heck of a place."

Tom was eyeing several young women who appeared to be in their early twenties. He swallowed the last of the pickle and said, "It's quite a place. Very remote. No one bothers me out there."

"It's not all that bad here, you know, Tom. Dad doesn't have the energy to be abusive any more. You should come back, we could use the help."

Tom gave Dan a friendly slap on the shoulder, took a last longing look at the women who, it seemed to him, were more interested in the other men around them and started towards the Harley.

"You're going?" Dan asked.

"Yeah," Tom said, "Thanks for bringing me, Dan, but I should be getting back. It's a long drive."

"It's early!" Dan said to the retreating figure.

"Getting supplies first!" Tom shouted from a distance back to Dan, "See you in a month or so!"

Tom started the motorcycle and made his way to the general store.

Tom parked the Harley in front of the store and dismounted. In front of the store stood a young woman leaning back in the sun against the brick wall. Tom looked at her, but she barely acknowledged him. She was wearing a light blue dress with clusters of faded flowers, probably made from a flour sack, and although it hung loose, the slim curves of her body were evident beneath it. She wore oxfords on her feet without socks, but in spite of her obvious poverty, she was strikingly pretty. Her blonde hair hung softly in curls around her face and reached below her shoulders. Her eyes were tired and hollow, but a bright and beautiful cornflower blue, and so strikingly deep and sad that Tom stared for several moments.

As she glanced toward Tom a second time, he could see that her skin was almost translucent and clear. She held a somewhat frazzled straw hat in her hands in front of her and shifted from one foot to the other with the opposite foot up against the wall in back.

She was waiting silently and expectantly, yet had an air of resignation about her. She looked sad to Tom.

He moved in her direction and smiled as he approached. "Hello," he said.

"'Lo," she said as she turned her full attention to him and gave him a crocked little smile that flickered for a moment and then was gone.

"My name's Tom, what's yours?"

Without enthusiasm she answered, "Anna."

Tom stood in front of her and a little to the side. He made a move towards the front door of the store, figuring that maybe she was a solitary soul, like himself, and probably wanted to be left alone. As he began to move, she spoke again.

"Nice motorcycle," she said with a slightly better attempt at a smile.

"Have you ever ridden one?" Tom asked. Then he said before she could answer, "I'll take you for a ride, if you would like."

Anna ventured a larger smile and walked toward Tom. "Where?" she asked.

"Around the block?" Tom said, "It doesn't have to be far – I promise to bring you right back."

Anna looked disappointed at this, but still accepted the offer and climbed onto the seat behind Tom. He started the Harley, and she clung tightly to him as they roared down a few streets, circled back and pulled up again at the general store. When he had shut the engine off, she still clung to him.

"It's OK to get off now," he said, worried that she was so afraid she couldn't move. Anna's body trembled slightly and she hung on tighter.

"Where do you live?" she asked him hesitantly.

Tom began to get suspicious; this girl seemed emotionally traumatized in some way, and it was evident that she was afraid to let go, but not for fear of falling off. It seemed as though she was afraid that he would drop her off here and leave her alone. Tom felt compassion, but he also didn't want trouble.

"I live out in the woods," he said, "Up the Appalachian Trail."

"Show me," she said.

"Anna, your family will miss you. I don't want you to get into trouble."

"They won't miss me," she said, "Believe me, no one here will know I'm even gone. Please, I want to go away from here."

Tom started the engine, and then shut it off again. "I'll take you, Anna, but first leave a message for your family. And tell them that you won't be back today. It takes too long to reach my place so I won't be bringing you back today. You'll have to spend the night."

Without a word, Anna jumped off the bike, ran into the store and exchanged words with the shopkeeper. Then she quickly reached behind the counter and retrieved a small pack tied with rope as a handle and placed it over her back. She ran back outside and climbed back on the motorcycle. Tom started the engine and they took the shortest road out of the town. By three o'clock in the afternoon they were rutting up the path to the cabin. Anna had screamed once or twice as they took some tight turns back on the country road, then she would laugh and spread her arms wide in the warm wind, laughing all the louder as she did. Tom smiled at this, but wondered why he was taking her with him; she was obviously a battered soul in some way.

Perhaps, he thought, I can find out what's hurting her and help. Tom had experience with troubles in his past. He didn't carry too much of a burden these days, but he could certainly read the signs. Anna was in trouble and he suspected she was homeless, or as close to that as you can get without actually having to live on the street.

When they bumped to a stop at the cabin, Anna stared around her in amazement. She slowly dismounted, and adjusting her dress back down around her knees, she looked back at Tom.

"This is all yours?" she asked.

Tom laughed, "No. Not really. It was abandoned, so I'm borrowing it for now."

Anna climbed the stairs and peered inside. While she was investigating, Tom covered the Harley and pushed it under the cabin. It was just starting to sprinkle so Tom quickly followed her up and invited her inside.

She sat down on his cot and watched as he lit the kerosene lantern. Piles of books were on the floor in disarray.

"Did you read all of these?" Anna asked.

"Almost," Tom said, "I'm getting low. I need to buy some more."

Anna found a book with the cover torn off; the first page said, "Collected works of Keats." She idly flipped through several pages while Tom watched.

"Anna," he said, and she looked up, "Anna, where is your family? Do you still live at home?"

Anna looked down quickly. She didn't meet his gaze when she murmured, "No. No, not really."

"Then how do you live?" Tom asked. She was silent and fingered the book in her lap. "Does your father beat you?" he asked, and then continued, "Anna, I can see you're in trouble. You shouldn't have come out here with me. It's probably not the right thing to do." Her eyes flared angrily, but he put his hand up to stop her.

"Come on, Anna, I'm glad you did, but I need to know more about you. I need to know why you wanted to get away so badly that you would just

59

accept a ride into the middle of nowhere with a stranger." Anna was quiet, and tears started to well in her eyes.

"I hate my life," she said, "You don't know…" She trailed off.

Tom came and sat beside her. He took her small hand in his and squeezed it slightly.

"Tell me," Tom said, "I won't think anything bad of you, I promise."

Anna looked up at Tom, then ahead at the lantern. It was throwing a soft glow around the cabin that flickered on the worn wooden boards across the room. In a rush of words, she poured out her life. Tom listened attentively to every word. His fears were realized when he discovered that she was fast becoming the town prostitute. Her aspiration had been to move to a larger city, as she was nearly starving in the small town, and she hoped to make more money in a metropolitan area. She would be gone, she said, as soon as she had the money for the bus ticket. Tom listened, then asked her about her family, and how she came to be in this situation. She started with her childhood…

Anna had a tough life right from the beginning. Her mother died in childbirth when she tried to deliver Anna's baby brother, who also died. The baby's cord had wrapped tightly around his neck. Her drunken father; taking the blue baby as a bad omen, proceeded to beat Anna's mother. Her mother soon bled to death.

The baby boy was buried along with her mother and that was that. Anna was just six years old at the time.

After that, her father expected her to do all the work that her mother had done before he had killed her, yet it was impossible for a six year old. There had been no school for Anna. Her father wouldn't let her go, and when she was only nine and he was drunk on corn liquor, as was his way every weekend, he raped her for the first time.

From then on she hid from him whenever the weekends came. She'd run away into the hills taking what little food she could find and her mother's old straw hat with the faded flowers on it. Her mother had worn it to church for as long as Anna could remember. It was one of the two cherished items that she had left to remember her by - the hat and her mother's family bible that had writing in the margins in her mother's own hand. She loved the very smell of both of them and would bury her head into her mother's hat just so she could try to remember what her mother smelled like. It always made her cry during those first hard years, but finally she could do it. She could just remember and not cry anymore, at least on the outside.

The woods became her place of solitude. A place to be safe from her father's constant ranting and ravings. He seemed to become more and more violent with the passing of time and she knew he hated her and blamed her for the death of her brother. He told her so directly in one of his drunken stupors. He had said that he never wanted "no dumb, no good, girl." And that it was her fault her brother was dead.

So, when her father would not notice her, she would take her blanket and a little food and go to a small cave she had found that was dry and fairly warm. She would wait it out until she knew her father was gone to work in the mines come Monday morning.

It was the way she survived the weekends. Then, when it was safe to return home on Monday, she'd creep back to their dilapidated house, and the cycle would start all over again.

As she got older, she tried to go to school. Her mother had told her about school many times – about how important it was and how much she'd like it, but that didn't work out very well. Most of the kids, even though from other poor families, were still far better off than she was. They shunned her and embarrassed her until she could not stand to attend the classes. All she could do to learn was to pick up the assignments after school when the other children had left for the day. She finally just gave up after she learned to read and write a little.

Most of her mother's family lived too far away to be of any help to Anna and so she grew up basically alone without friends or family.

When she was fifteen years old, one of her father's drunken friends caught her alone in the house one day when he was looking for her dad. By the time she recognized the look in his eye, it was too late. He forced her into the bedroom where he raped her.

After it was over, he tossed a dollar on her chest and said, "Thanks." She spit at him and tore the dollar up, but it gave her an idea. If men were so eager to be with her, had such strong and urgent desires, then why not make them pay. She recognized this as a possible escape from the misery of this place.

She tried it out in town a few days later hanging around the outside of a bar where the miners and farmers frequented. She didn't know anyone and so she was able to pretend she was just waiting for someone until the right looking man appeared. It didn't take long and her destiny was soon sealed.

Tom listened without comment. Inside he felt a revulsion and hatred for

Anna's father, but he kept his expression neutral. When Anna had finished, Tom gently wiped a tear off her face, and struggling to keep his voice calm, he said, "Never mind all that now, Anna. It's over. It's *your* life now, and you can do whatever you want to with it." Anna turned and hugged Tom. She shook softly as she cried silently. Tom felt his own hot tears on his cheeks, and he whispered to her that it would all be all right. He held her that way for a half an hour, and when she was calmed, he gently pulled her arms from his neck, walked over and started his small camp stove.

While he waited for a can of stew to heat, he opened the poetry book and read some sonnets to Anna. She listened and watched him. He would read a poem, and then ask her if she felt anything about the words.

"I don't understand them," she would confess with honesty, "They're pretty words, but I don't know what they're trying to say." Tom would go back over a part of the poem and explain it to her with infinite patience. Occasionally, her face would light up, and she would smile and interject. Tom watched her and was happy that she was, at least for the moment, distracted. He read several more poems and then attended to dinner. He prepared two bowls of stew and garnished them with some small carrots he had grown nearby. Anna ate hungrily and watched Tom the entire time, her eyes never leaving him. When she had nearly eaten the entire serving, she stopped and placed the plate on the floor.

She looked at Tom and asked, "Are you a teacher, Tom? You must be because you read all these books. Did you go to college to learn these things?"

Tom smiled, "No, not a teacher, in fact I didn't really go to college either, except for a while to learn Japanese."

"You speak Japanese?" she asked incredulously, "Say something to me."

Tom cleared his throat, then said,

> *"Asagao no*
> *Hanada no*
> *awaki Inochi oshi."*

Anna's eyes were wide. "What did you say?" she said.

Tom gave the classic Haiku poem to her in English, "It means, more or less,

I love the rest of my life
Though it is transitory
Like a light azure morning glory."

"What's azure?" Anna asked.

"It's a color, sort of blue, I think," Tom answered.

"Do you really love your life?" Anna asked.

"I didn't write the poem," Tom said.

"But," Anna persisted, "Do you love your life?"

Tom sighed. He collected the dishes and set them by the doorway and turned back to Anna.

"I don't know," he said finally. Anna seemed satisfied with the answer and laid down on the cot. Tom watched her, and then laid down next to her. They watched the stars come out through the opening.

After about an hour, Anna said, "Write me a poem."

"Sure," Tom said, "I'll try to write one about you…it'll be a poem about a girl who wants to travel. She'll be afraid, but she will go away one day and find a happy place, far from her past. I think she'll find out at some point that she is really a princess that has been kept in a prison, but once free, she'll learn to fly like the birds."

"Yes," Anna said, "Write that one." With that, she fell fast asleep, and Tom listened to the quiet sounds of the night.

Tom didn't sleep much that night. He spent most of the night thinking about Anna and his own life.

Morning was bright and warm after the rain. The air was clear and clean and Tom put the coffee pot on to heat the water, then walked down to the river to look at the tracks left during the night by all the little animals. Anna was still sleeping, but stirred when Tom climbed the stairs. He started breakfast cooking and the smell of bacon rose up through the open windows. Coffee was perking in an old aluminum pot.

Anna sat up with a start and looked around as if she didn't know where she was, then seeing Tom, she relaxed.

"Eat some breakfast," he said, "and then I have to take you back."

She washed in the stone cistern outside and then ran back up the stairs.

"That smells really good, thanks, Tom."

She asked him if he had finished his poem about her.

Tom laughed, "No, Anna! It takes time, I need to think about it for a while."

"When will it be done?" she asked in her innocent, but direct manner. "Can I come back and hear it when you've finished?"

"I'll take you home, and then if everything's OK, I'll pick you back up in a week. Maybe by then I'll have completed it." Tom paused in thought, and then said, "Anna, you can make something of your life, you know." He took her small hand in his. "Despite your past and all the pain, you still can make something of yourself. You're pretty, and smart. I know because you can understand some things that a lot of people can't understand. You only have to find a way to change your situation and then…you can become anything you want to be."

Anna listened, then said, "Then what about you, Tom? Are you making something of your life here? Yes, it's pretty, but is this *all* you want out of your life? You keep on tellin' me that I can do so much, but what about you? You're hiding from life, just like me."

Anna finished, immediately regretted it and apologized. "I'm sorry. You're so nice and kind. I shouldn't even compare us."

Tom was angry at first, but saw her remorse and felt saddened. "No, Anna, it's OK. You have a point," he said, "I am hiding from life."

"I'm sorry," she said again. She collected her things and waited for Tom to pull the Harley out from under the corncrib cabin and start it.

They mounted the motorcycle and drove back to town. When Tom dropped her off, she gave him a quick kiss on the cheek.

"I'll be here waiting for you in one week," she said.

Tom took her hand, kissed it lightly and said, "I'll be back then." And he rode off.

One week later, Tom pulled into town and found Anna waiting at the storefront. She smiled and waved. She was holding a package that she could barely carry.

"I bought something for you," she said.

"You bought something?" Tom asked, "What? And why?" He didn't want to ask her how.

"Books!" Anna said with excitement. She opened the bag and inside there were several books on philosophy. "I know how much you like to think, Tom, so I found these for you. I don't know what they are or what they say, but I knew you would."

Tom pulled one out. "Existentialism, from Descartes to Hume" it read.

Tom smiled and stowed the assortment into a saddlebag.

"Thanks, Anna."

When they were back at the cabin, Tom unpacked and Anna unloaded her few belongings.

"I've been thinking," she said, and then as Tom looked her way, she continued, "I've been thinking about what you said last week."

Tom waited and she finished, "And I think that you're right. I can make something of my life and I am going to. But…I think you should have to do something too."

"And what's that, Anna?" Tom said.

"I think you need to be a teacher, Tom. I think you need to teach because you're good and so smart. It would be a waste for you to spend the rest of your life out here alone."

Tom watched her and smiled, but said, "I'd have to go to college first. I'm not qualified to teach anything right now."

"But you could!" Anna said, "You could go to college. I heard some soldiers talk about it. They say that after the war, the government pays for college, so you could go!"

Tom laughed. It *was* a thought. Certainly, this was not the ultimate use of his time.

"I guess you're right, Anna. Maybe I should consider that. Maybe I can go, but if I do, you have to promise me something. You have to promise that you'll quit prostitution and get a job as a waitress or something. And then you have to promise that you'll find a man, but not a man like your dad. He'll have to be a man that's kind to you. Promise?"

Anna looked at Tom and realized that he was just such a man, but at the same time, he was inviting her to move on away from him and onto something better and attainable.

She wanted Tom, but she also realized that he wasn't available.

"Will you let me stay here for awhile?" she asked, "I want to stay for a week or two, and then I'll leave. I promise I'll do those things, but only if you promise too." She smiled at him and he almost became lost in the beauty of her eyes, so alive now and so different from the first time he had seen her. But he knew it would be the wrong thing for both of them.

Anna stayed with Tom for two weeks. They walked the trails around the cabin, sometimes in light rain, and sometimes in downpours. She clung to Tom when they crossed slippery rocks, and she listened to his every word.

On the final day, she recited a poem she had thought up, the first attempt she had ever made at any such thing. It was simple, yet deep in emotion. It spoke of a mountain man, who longed for the sun, but locked himself away in a cave of darkness. Tom listened, and then recited his poem to Anna. She cried when he finished.

Tom dropped her off in the town near the café. She said she had business there. She was going to work for them, at first for free if she had to. She assured Tom that her life was changed. She was going to work at a regular job, and then, if things went well, she was going to go to school. She held her mother's old torn straw hat in one hand and carried her Bible in a brown paper sack, the two most precious things she owned along with Tom's poem.

Tom kissed her goodbye, and then headed back to the cabin. He stood in the middle of his 'home' and looked around. It held good memories for him, probably the best he had ever had, but it was time to leave.

He wrote a quick note to whoever might chance upon the place, that there was a fine carrot patch one hundred yards northeast, and if the rabbits had not devastated it, the carrots were exceptionally sweet. He left the bulk of the books. It would take too many trips to take them all back. He scrawled a note and stuck it in the wall over the stacks. "Walden Library" it said. He tucked an application to the University of West Virginia in his pocket, along with an application for the G.I. bill and headed home.

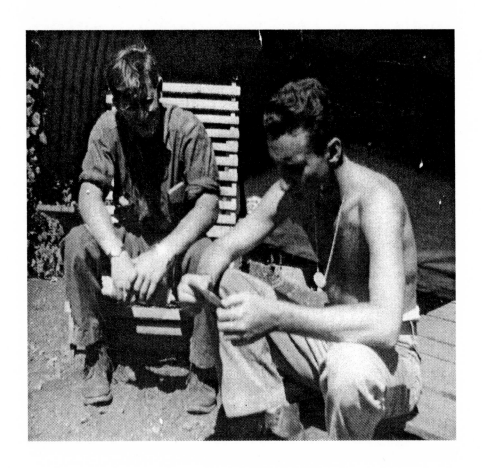

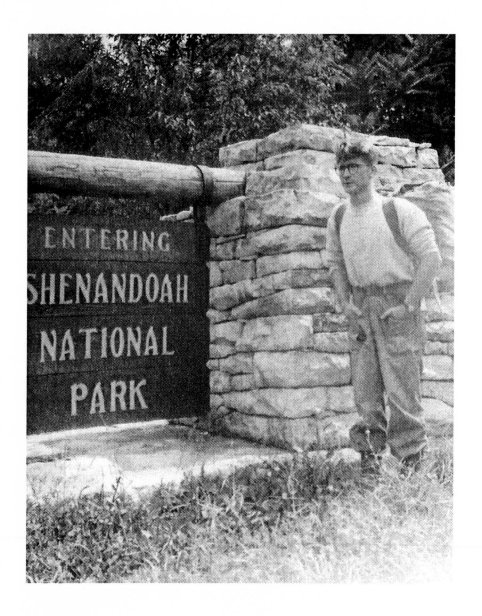

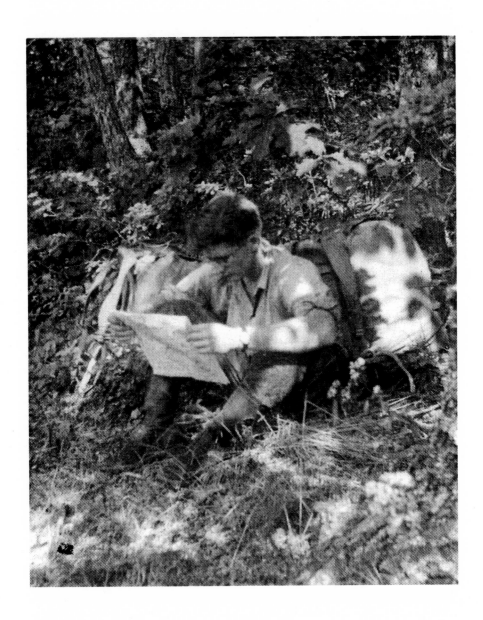

Chapter Five

Watchers of the stars - suggest a master cistern, spawning bed of time…

Janice was concerned over homosexuality. Not for herself, she was happily married, but for her brother who was making the overtures of "coming out of the closet." This really disturbed Janice since she loved her brother, and yet like the rest of her family, she was horrified over the situation. Janice's family, like many Americans, ranged from devout Christian to a more ecumenical, but still generally religious, attitude.

As Janice's brother was wrestling with his conscience, the family was wrestling in debate. Mack, the father, grew red faced and refused to discuss the situation. Jana, the mother, was compassionate, but wanted desperately for her son to reconsider. She was certain that her son was just a little confused. All he needed was to find the right girl, and his fascination for boys would be swept away like the dead leaves she swept off the front porch each evening.

Janice stood on the fence with regard to the whole issue. It seemed to her that her mother had a good point, but when she spoke through teary eyes with Jason, she gradually came to accept the fact that this was not something that would go away as easily as eucalyptus leaves.

The debate centered over whether or not being gay is something ingrained within the person, or if being gay is something that is a matter of choice. In this day and age (1985), there was still considerable persecution of the gay community. Janice grieved and worried over her little brothers' future. She had a vivid picture of the suffering he might endure.

She wanted to change him if she could, but she was determined to know the truth. Could it be a matter of choice? Is it something brought on by a reaction to an overbearing father or mother? Is this, she pondered, something influenced by society and the pressures it places on certain young boys?

It was important to Janice to understand and to know the nature of the matter, and because of that, she brought the topic up frequently at work in the dental office.

As unusual as it might seem, this dental office held many such discussions.

70

The pace here was slow and we had learned, unexpectedly, that rural American families carried a myriad of problems with them far beyond the scope of fillings and root canals. It was shocking, at first, to hear confessions from a middle-aged woman in the dental chair as she elaborated on her family life. Often these elaborations included personal problems regarding her husband, her children or the abuse she suffered as a child. Frequently the careful, studied comments of 'hmm' and 'I see' were masking our shock at the full disclosures everyday patients offered without reservation.

So, as Janice brought the discussion with her into "Operatory One" and continued to ask for guidance and/or insight, I carried along with her, to a degree, and acted as a conduit for her emotional distress.

We were about to examine a new patient, and this white haired, grizzled older man who rode in on a motorcycle in full leathers was unlikely (in our minds) to object. The patient, Tom Law, as his medical chart told us, was in for a routine exam. As I perused his chart, Janice concluded with the final and essential question, "So, do you think my brother has a choice in the matter?"

Turning my attention away from my examination of the chart, I looked back to Janice with an, "I don't know, but feel your frustration" look.

Our patient, who had been quietly listening, cleared his throat and spoke, "I can induce it in rats,", he calmly said.

"I beg your pardon?" I said, "Rats?"

"Yes, in rats," he continued, "During the first week, which is equivalent to the first trimester in humans, on the fourth day, a minor…very minor…fluctuation in estrogen in the pregnant female will make her male young homosexual. In fact, they will not only be homosexual, but they will exhibit all of the characteristic behaviors of female rats, including nurturing of the young, picking them up and carrying the infant rats that have strayed, right back to the nest. Behaviors only exhibited in typical female rats."

Janice came alive. "Are you saying, Tom,"

"Doctor Law," I corrected.

"Are you saying, *Doctor* Law, that *Humans* are homosexual because of something that happens to them during pregnancy?"

"Yes," he continued, "humans have the same hormones as rats and other animals. And just as I have induced it in laboratory animals, fluctuations in estrogen occur occasionally in a human, which, if it happens exactly at the right time, causes homosexuality. It isn't a choice for the infant male. When he reaches puberty, he will be gay."

71

Janice was quiet, but I noticed a small smile at the corners of her mouth. She was thinking, and she realized that she now had some tools to use in her family crisis. I was smiling too, but not for the same reason. I had perceived this patient to be similar to some of the fishermen that frequented my practice. They usually called on the emergency line with toothaches, and while faithful in paying their bills, they rarely returned for routine treatments. A point that irritated me since I was frequently aroused out of a deep sleep to extract an infected tooth in the middle of the night. The fishermen were always gracious and appreciative, but a little preventative maintenance would have gone a long way.

This person, however, took me by surprise. His unkempt look notwithstanding, he had some credentials, that if true, belied an intelligence that we rarely encountered in this practice. I decided that I should learn a little more, so while Janice was taking a set of x-rays, I caught up with my schedule and considered what I wanted to ask Dr. Law.

When I returned to the operatory, Tom was sitting quietly, facing the painting of a duck that I had acquired in a trade with a local artist in exchange for dental work.

"The x-rays should be out soon," I said.

"Fine," Tom responded.

"Do you have any problems with your teeth?" I continued.

"No," Tom said, "I'm just in for a routine check."

"Where was your last dentist?" I asked.

"Mexico," Tom replied.

"How long were you in Mexico?" I asked.

"About ten years, give or take," Tom said, "…sailing."

"You are retired?" I asked.

"Yes," Tom replied.

"You were a Neurophysiologist?" I asked.

"Yes."

"Where?"

"Oh, a couple of places," Tom said, "I taught in the Medical School at the University of Michigan for some years, then later taught at Claremont University."

"Neurophysiology?" I pressed.

Tom chuckled, then said "Yes, more or less, but with a point."

Just then the x-rays arrived, and I turned my attention to them for several minutes. "I don't see any problems, but I think I'll schedule you with my hygienist for a cleaning," I said.

"OK," Tom replied.

I sat for a few moments contemplating this interesting man, as I moved some of my equipment and washed my hands.

"You mentioned you taught Neurophysiology, but with a 'point'" I said, smiling. "I'm just curious – what was that 'point'?"

Tom contemplated a moment, then replied, "Well," he said as he ran his fingers across the front of his graying hair, "Everything we do in life has a point, Dr. Norby."

"Call me Steve," I said, "All of my patients do here."

"OK, Steve," Tom continued, "I was saying that there are reasons to study and teach neurophysiology, besides the obvious surface points. We may not consciously know what the point is, or we may elect to hide if from our open acknowledgement, but if you care to dig deep enough, you find there are always reasons. I had mine. From the time I was a child I wanted to know what makes the human race tick. Why do we do the things we do? What is the logic behind our actions and thoughts? Or, if there isn't a logic to a certain action, then why do we take those actions?"

"I see," I said, and then went on, "But in reality, I had always thought that motivational behavior was the arena of psychology, or sociology. I would never have placed any importance in understanding humans in the field of physiology."

Tom smiled and said, "Neither would anyone else. I started my journey in Psychology, and I rapidly grew tired of that field. I wanted facts, and there are fundamental conflicts and contradictions in that discipline. Plus, to be honest, there was no future for me there. If I intended to make my mark in science, it would not be on the coat tails of the Icons of Psychology. Original theories were long since used up. Not to mention the fact that they were inherently wrong."

"Modern Psychology is *wrong?*" I asked.

"Modern Psychology has helped a great many people," Tom replied, "but it doesn't answer the most fundamental questions. For example, have you ever noticed that two *completely* different psychological approaches to the same type of patient can work?"

"Yes, I have noticed that there are a multitude of approaches to the same problem," I replied, "and also that the results don't seem as consistent as, say, prescribing an antibiotic that works every single time against a certain bacterium."

"Exactly," Tom said, "Sometimes a 'therapy' works in a situation, and the next time it doesn't."

"But why?" I asked.

"Because," Tom continued, "they're treating the brain as though it's modeling clay – a thing that started out as a smooth, round ball at birth and then became molded over time into the adult. To a large degree, the psychologists completely ignore the fact that the brain is like a computer – or at least they used to. You can write programs on it, but the hardware is everything, and the hardware has a certain way of functioning that determines what programs will work. The human brain, Steve, is every bit as hard-wired as a computer – maybe even more so."

I thought about this for a moment, and then I noticed that my allotted time was running out. Even in a relatively slow practice such as mine, I could only get away with just so much socializing. But I was intrigued. This person seemed very certain of something. It was very interesting and I was more than a little curious.

Perhaps it was due to the fact that teaching people how to brush and floss their teeth over so many years starves the dentist of intellectual stimulation, or perhaps it was simply that Tom was, in a way that I could not quite fathom at that time, different. But either way, I wanted to hear more, so at the risk of annoying my next patient, I decided to throw caution to the wind and continue. "So what did you do?" I asked, "How did you proceed in your career, and how did you prove your theories to be correct?"

"Well, at the time," Tom said, "everyone was studying and was completely engrossed in the theory called the 'neural mechanisms of learning', or in other words, the concept that we are psychologically a blank piece of paper at birth. In those days everyone was dedicated to proving that most, if not all, human behavior is learned and that the ability to learn so readily is what separates us from the other species."

"But you disagreed?" I said.

"Well, I was at least willing to *consider* it!" Tom smiled. "In those days it was sacrilege to suggest such a thing. The predominant belief was that man's unquestioned 'uniqueness' was entirely the result of a brain, and that this brain was a *blank slate* at birth. It was only later that science and music and culture and genius came into the picture. It was obvious, they proposed, that if all intelligence, wit and thought were written on a blank sheet by our experiences, then learning was the central mode by which all things came about, and so it had to be that man was the superior learner of the universe.

They did this, not so much to search out and find truth, but for the purpose of proving the superiority of 'Homo Sapiens.' It was, and still is, an approach born of the need to separate us from the other species on the planet. We humans have always had this need, and scientists are no different."

Tom sighed and continued, "Remember that early astronomers were imprisoned for suggesting that the Universe did not revolve around the Earth. Religions abounded with the concept that we are the very center of God's attention. Regardless of what may or may not be true, the fact is that it is an emotional need for humans to feel they are special or unique."

"But," I interjected, "aren't we unique? Isn't it obvious that we've accomplished things that no other species could possibly accomplish?"

Tom chuckled, and then said, "Of *course* we are unique! We are spectacular! But the fundamental key to understanding why is not to be found in 'learning', as the behaviorists would have us believe. We learn the same way that any other animal learns. Learning is characteristic of the lowest forms of life. A case can be made that even preliving forms learn. And where learning occurs, up and down the evolutionary scale from man to worm to germ, the form of the function is the same: a negatively accelerated, positive exponential curve."

"You lost me there...an exponential curve?" I asked.

"We learn the same way the flatworm does, in other words. Or the way any creature, even the simplest ones, learn," Tom answered.

"So what then, is so unique about that?" I asked.

"What indeed," Tom replied, "There is nothing all that unique, and that's why they couldn't stand the thought. There is nothing all that extraordinary about the way we learn. Every animal has the same constraints. Learn quickly what you need to know or die. There are too many predators out there, too many competitors, to make learning a leisurely process. That isn't what makes us Homo Sapiens unique. We learn quickly, Steve, of that there is no doubt. But so do monkeys and insects.

What makes us so successful is the fact that most of our advantage in this world, the thing that makes us dominant over everything, is that the *learning* was done a long time ago. We are the recipients of that glorious work. We have layers upon layers of brain matter that are built upon millennia."

"You are suggesting then, that this *information* is genetic?" I asked.

"More than you can imagine," Tom replied, "That was the essence of my research. I proved that human behavior is largely genetic."

I was not exactly happy to hear what Tom was saying. At this point. I still had over sixty thousand dollars in student loans to repay and the eight years of 'higher education' had been a great sacrifice to me. I doubted that any flat worm could have done it. I expressed this to Tom.

"You're missing the point, Steve," Tom replied, "Do you think that language is entirely learned?"

"Of course I do," I replied.

"Then how long, for example, do you think it would take you to learn a new one, say Spanish?" Tom asked.

"Well," I answered, "I guess if I were dedicated, it would take about a year or so."

"Then consider this," Tom continued, "You have a fully formed human brain. A brain that does not even reach its full size until the teen years, and yet an infant learns language in the first few years, and it does so without formal training. It happens in spite of the obvious fact that there are no classes on grammar and syntax, and the infant's brain is a fraction of the size it will be later in life. It's fair to say, I think, that the infant could not learn Dentistry, yet language, something challenging enough to take a year to learn, is accomplished in the early years by children."

He continued, "As if that were not obvious enough, there have been recent studies that show that language is 'programmed' into us. Even isolated people with no exposure will create a language. The fundamentals of the grammar and syntax will be consistent with all the major world languages. It's hard wired. It's a part of the brain that has been genetically preserved and passed on. It has nothing to do with a blank slate."

"So your research was aimed in this direction?" I asked, "You were focused on how language is 'hard wired' in the human brain?"

"Yes and no," Tom replied, "My research was focused on the brain, and the mechanisms that were present as a part of the hardware, but when I began, it was the core of the brain that I focused on. The core is the chassis upon which everything else is built. It's the engine, the drive train and the fuel, all at once. Language and other preestablished programs are written over that."

Tom looked at Steve and pushed his hair off his forehead.

"The basis of everything, Steve, was to be found in the Hypothalamus. It's there that the fundamental drive that propels us through life is found. The drive that, for lack of a better word, you could call instinct."

"You mean the drive for survival?" I asked.

"Nope," Tom replied, "The drive for procreation – the sexual drive, that's above everything else. It is the most powerful drive we have."

"That sounds a bit Freudian, if I may say so," I commented, "Yet you're against psychology and it's precepts, so why the focus on sexuality? How can that be more important than survival?"

Tom laughed again, and then said, "Would you believe that a father or mother of a child would give their life to save the child?"

"Yes," I answered, "I'm certain that most parents would give their life to save their child."

"Then what's more important, the person's life or the life of their child?" Tom asked.

Obviously, the life of their child." I responded.

"And how do we make children?" Tom asked.

"Via sex," I responded, "but we're talking about survival here, not sex. How do you equate the two?"

"It's simple," Tom said, "We don't have children without sex, at least not until very recently, and the program is built in layers. Layer one is the drive to have children, i.e. sex. Layer two is to preserve those children. Layer three is to survive personally, and so on."

"So," I continued in disbelief, "You're saying that the basic programs of the brain are built upon a sexual drive?"

"I proved it." Tom said, "I created the original probe that mapped every portion of the brain and demonstrated the functions. It was controversial, especially then, to understate the fact. Ultimately, it cost me my career. Yet the facts are most certainly there. The neurotransmitters that control our emotions, our thoughts and our behavior are fundamentally linked to the chassis of the brain, and the function of that chassis is procreation."

I looked at Tom for a moment and considered what he was saying. In many ways, it was revolting. I liked to think that humans were highly evolved beings, complete with Divine essence and a higher calling. What he was proposing was that we are a basic life form, similar to other animals. My mind raced from images of dogs in heat to the tabloids on grocery store counters, and I didn't like the comparison. Yet the image was there, and I couldn't deny that much of our entertainment media pandered to base desires. How, I wondered, would these sitcoms exist if not for the fact that we, as humans, were intently focused on such things? How *intrinsic* was this drive? Tom's logic was irritating, and he seemed completely smug with his statements. I was not comfortable, but I was also a scientist by nature, and I wanted to know more. Perhaps, I thought, I could find holes in his theories.

At the very least, I determined to contemplate his statements and come up with my own questions and theories.

Throughout these reflections, I came back to the fact that Tom was my patient, and I needed to attend to him.

He had opened up considerably in this first visit, and I honored that in a person, and so I continued with a few more questions.

"You mentioned that your research was controversial and that it cost you your career?" I asked, "I can't imagine what happened."

"As I said," Tom continued, "No one in that day and age tolerated the possibility of instinctual behavior and sex was literally unmentionable. If you mentioned it, you would definitely be shouted out of a seminar or patronized as mentally handicapped for suggesting that instinct played a role in our lives, and...no scientist mentioned sex at all. Incredibly, they would rather take the position that sex was learned than drop their fantasy that *all* human behavior was *free* of instinct. If they were forced to refer to sex at all, it was in cocktail lounges at conventions."

"They couldn't accept that sexual behavior has a basis in instinct?" I asked.

"Exactly," Tom said, "Remember, this was decades ago, and the prudery was something paramount to the Puritans who founded this nation. So at the least I had the whole field to myself!"

"But," I said, "You knew that there would be hell to pay for going against the grain."

Tom contemplated my remark for a few moments. "Yes..." he commented, "It was against the grain, and I went that direction with what I now can see was reckless abandon. I reasoned that my studies would be controversial and funding would be very difficult to gain. But think about it, the whole of the world was my laboratory. When it comes right down to it, who needs money to study sex? I knew that there would be challenges in publishing any findings. I knew that garnering graduate students to help with the research would be problematic since they would be aligning themselves with a pariah, but I also knew that I was on the right track."

Janice entered the room and gave me an irritated look. I had taken too much time with this patient and needed to get back to work. I needed a break as well. Tom's postulations were disturbing and the thought of a simple exam or filling was a relief. I excused myself from Tom, but asked him a question before I left.

"I'm really interested in your career and how it turned out," I said, "Would you be willing to tell me more about it the next time you come in?"

Tom looked up from the dental chair with a look of mixed emotions. "I can tell you," he said, "But it's not a happy story. There's not a lot of support for my theories and most people don't want to hear them."

"I do," I said with a smile as I shook his hand, "I'll see you next time."

I left the operatory and greeted my next patient. Happily, it was a child in for a small filling. It was routine and the child was cooperative, which freed my mind to wander for a few brief moments. I was anxious to see Tom again and continue the discussion.

Chapter Six

What auditor of the endless spheres
cast this secret stone to the farthest pond
past the grasp of hope and yearning?

Tom didn't return to my office for several months, and in the interim I pondered his statements about human sexuality. If I was squeamish about it, I could readily see how his contemporaries might have felt decades ago. Television programming had changed just since I was a child, and the first radio announcer to use a distasteful word had been fired from his job. The first time the word "damn" was used in the cinema was in the movie, "Gone With The Wind", and it created quite a ruckus. Yet now, the culture of our nation had changed. Skirting the issue at first, and then closing in ever nearer, the media that surrounded us seemed intent on a sexual theme. Since the media responded to consumer demand, I reasoned, there was validation in Tom's precept that we humans are very interested in sex. I was surprised, but not deeply. If you took the time to look around, you came to the inescapable conclusion that, like it or not, we were tuning into the shows on TV or reading tabloids that offered glimpses into sexual behavior.

Tom's career must have been exciting, even if it didn't end in a pleasant manner.

I was happy to see him when he returned, and I asked him to tell me about his research. Fortunately for the routine of the dental office, I had him scheduled just prior to a two hour lunch in the anticipation of the wrath of Janice.

When I completed repairing the small chip on one of his front teeth, I dismissed Janice from her duties and asked Tom to tell me about his teaching.

I sat his chair back up and since it was comfortable for him, we decided to visit right there in the operatory. I hadn't realized until that moment just how anxious I was to speak with this learned professor. Something about him intrigued me.

He looked at me and smiled, brushed the hair from his forehead and said, "I started teaching at the University of Michigan," Tom began, "But that was years after I had been enrolled there."

"You were a student at Michigan?" I asked.

"Yes, I transferred there from West Virginia," Tom said, "As a psychology major."

"Were you studying sexuality then?" I asked.

Tom laughed. "Oh sure! I was studying it on my own time!" he exclaimed, "I was a student, and like the rest of the young men, I was intent on dating whenever possible. In fact, perhaps my later interest in sexuality came about as a result of my failures in that department."

I laughed and said, "Tell me about that!"

Tom settled into his chair and reflected. I glanced at the clock, lots of time left, I thought. Lunch would have to be taken later, if at all.

"My roommate and I decided to learn to sail on Lake Michigan," Tom began, "Partly because it would be a fun diversion, and partly because we both had independently come to the conclusion that a boat would be a surefire way to impress the ladies. Actually, my roommate was already an accomplished sailor. His father had run contraband in the North Sea during the First World War. The contraband boat was similar to an old pirate ship, complete with black sails, and though he never confessed it, I suspected that his father had been running munitions. At any rate, my roommate and I scraped enough cash together to purchase an old catboat. It was decrepit, but it sailed well enough. The trouble was we couldn't afford to store it or pay docking fees, so we came up with the brilliant notion to sink it with rocks by the shore whenever we were done with it for the day. It worked beautifully. On the days that we were not in classes or studying for exams, we would hitch a ride to the lake and wade in the cold water to our vessel. Once we lifted out the rocks, it was a matter of minutes before we had it bailed out and floating. The sail we retrieved from its hiding place buried under brush, and off we would go. Before long, I felt proficient enough to launch my plan.

There was a girl that I had been courting. I was able to convince her to come to the lake and take a sail on the beautiful blue waters. A lot of planning went into my preparations. I had packed a picnic basket with lunch and drinks. I had even made a trip to the lake beforehand to lift the boat and towel it off inside. I wanted everything to go smoothly, but as usual, that was never the case.

My date and I arrived at the beach, and with a flourish, I helped her into the boat and we shoved off. It was a beautiful day, and my plan was proceeding perfectly. Errol Flynn, I was, on the open sea with a lovely lady. It would just be a matter of time I felt, before she would succumb to my charms." Tom was chuckling in earnest now as he related the story.

I asked him if he was comfortable and he said he was, so I grabbed a couple of cups of hot tea and hurried back into the operatory so he could continue. Tom took a sip of his tea and then picked up where he had left off.

"Everything was progressing fine in our sailing, until suddenly the wind stopped. Completely."

"Really?" I asked.

"Yes! No one had ever told me, but on Lake Michigan, most evenings the wind stops at about 6:00 pm. Without the wind, we were stranded. It was getting cold and dark and the young lady was becoming ever more unhappy. Even the delicacies I had provided in the basket did little to please her. So there we were, a good distance from the shore, cold, and no wind at all!" Tom shook his head in disbelief at his own predicament.

"There was a single oar on the boat, and I began the long paddle towards the bank. We arrived just as the sun was rising, and though it was a beautiful sight, the young lady didn't seem to share my enthusiasm. She left in a huff and I never saw her again."

I laughed at Tom's mishap. "Did you ever have any success with the boat?" I asked.

"Never," Tom replied, "It was always the same. I never got anywhere, no matter how hard I tried. You would have thought that I'd have figured out that sailing, in order to impress the ladies, just might not be the way to go, but I doggedly kept at it. I kept falling on my nose in the female department. I would get up and try again, but always with the same results! The worst, the absolute worst time, was when I was sailing with a girl I really had fallen for, and it started to get stormy. Storms on Lake Michigan can crop up instantly, and that's what happened this time. One minute it was beautiful, with just enough wind to show my expertise as captain of my vessel, and I was just beginning to believe that this girl was duly impressed, then the next minute we were fighting white caps and high winds. Fortunately, we weren't that far out, and I thought to be chivalrous by placing my coat over her shoulders and grinning in false confidence as I labored to get us to shore. We were getting close to making it, but then I looked back and saw a giant wave headed for us. I knew it would catch us and we would no doubt capsize, which could really hurt someone if they were hit on the head by the boom or mast.

So I made a quick decision, one that I would later live to regret. I yelled, 'Quick! Jump for your life! A tidal wave is coming at us!' And with that I jumped into the water.

Now in my defense, I expected her to follow suit, but she didn't. She sort of got up and made a half jump for the side, then sat half way back down." Tom laughed at the predicament.

"I was fully in the water now and bobbing around looking in utter fascination at her hanging on for dear life as the huge wave approached. The wave struck the back quarter of the boat, but it didn't tumble. Rather, it and its occupant, were completely swamped in a gurgling froth of cold water.

That girl got off the boat in such a manner and in such a wet hurry that I simply stood there in the water, amazed. She was drenched from her head, to her soggy, wet shoes and mad! Oh my! She was mad! She didn't even push her hair out of her face, you know, like most women do. She just stomped and sloshed right on by me murmuring bad things about my genealogy as she proceeded straight up to her car. Fortunately for her, she had hidden her key. Unfortunately for me, I had no way home. It was after I sank the boat with rocks that I was faced with a long trek back. I never saw her again, and come to think of it, she never returned my jacket."

I had begun laughing at the first indication of where this story was going and could hardly contain myself at the end.

"So this was your introduction to the Science of Human Sexuality?" I asked, laughing still.

Tom smiled, and then became more serious. "No, not really," he said, "But I'm sure it contributed. Every male wants to know what a female is looking for so that he can increase his odds, and every female wants similar knowledge. Certainly I had personal interest, but my career in that arena happened as an accident, really."

"You didn't start your research in that area?" I asked.

"No," Tom replied, "No, I was a student, remember, so I did what I was told to do. And much of what was interesting or vital knowledge in those days was banned."

"How so?" I asked.

"The study of 'reproduction' was at the time limited to sea urchins, and if you happened to be in a very liberal college, you might study rats without getting into trouble. But anything more advanced than that and you were asking for trouble."

"I remember trying to fertilize a sea urchin egg in zoology lab," I offered.

"Yes. Well, they're large eggs and easy to work with, which is why they're used. But the problem is not in the fundamental aspects of the procedure, it is in the perception of lascivious conduct. That's what holds everyone back."

"I take it you went beyond rats," I said.

"Eventually," Tom said, "I did eventually."

"I'd love to hear that story," I said, "Would you be willing to tell it to me? I'm interested."

"Sure, be happy to. I'll tell you," Tom said, "But it'll take some time. Maybe we should meet to discuss it when you don't have any interruptions?" Tom politely asked.

"Tomorrow?" I said. "I'll meet you at the coffee house tomorrow, and if it is OK, I would like to record this. I think it is very interesting, and I want to be able to go over it later."

"I'll see you then," Tom said.

I arranged to meet Tom at five o'clock the following day, and with my tape recorder in hand, I asked him to start from the beginning. It was a beginning that started in undergraduate school...

Tom stood on the curb where the bus had dropped him off and looked long and hard at the entry to the University. It was vast and ancient, completely different from the University of West Virginia where he had just attended. The University of Michigan was well known. West Virginia was a flyspeck in those days. He had been more or less shoved out the door at West Virginia. They were all smiles and congratulatory back there, but he knew that they were relieved to be rid of him.

They transferred him to Michigan, practically filling out the applications for him. He could imagine both the faculty and administration were probably holding a party this very minute.

Not that he hadn't been a good student, per se; he was the most brilliant student the West Virginia faculty had probably ever seen. But he had a way of being very direct and challenging, a way not always appreciated by his professors.

When he began his first semester at college, his brilliance came as much of a surprise to him as it did to everyone else. He knew that he was intelligent, but he naturally expected college students and the professors to be as much or more intelligent than himself. That had been his first disappointment with college. The students he could accept, after all, they were the ones paying to learn. But his professors back at West Virginia fell far below his expectations.

Well, he surmised, here at Michigan it would be different. This would be the place where brilliance lived, where his mind would be challenged. Maybe here, he would find the answers to the questions that had been haunting him for years.

Tom shuffled onto campus and found the library. Making a mental note of its location, he asked passers by until he found the student housing office. He plopped his duffle bag on the floor in front of a bulletin board and scanned the tacked up notes until he had the names of three students seeking roommates. With their phone numbers scribbled on a scrap of paper, he hoisted his duffle, found a pay phone and dialed the first one.

"Hello?" answered a male voice on the other end.

"I found your notice that you're looking for a roommate. Is the room still available?" Tom asked.

"Are you a freshman?" asked the voice on the other end of the line.

"Junior," Tom answered, "Transferred from West Virginia."

"Bio Major?" the voice probed.

Tom grimaced inside. He was, in fact, in the psychology department and embarrassed by the fact. More and more he had begun to feel like the answers he sought would not be found in this nebulous field, but still, he was constrained to stick it out. It wasn't *real* science in his mind, but he had a notion of where it could take him later.

"Psychology," he answered flatly.

There was a pause, then, "Me too. Come on over. You know how to get here?"

"I have your address," Tom said, "I'll be right there." The line clicked on the other end, and Tom shouldered the duffle and headed back towards the library.

The ancient house was only a few blocks removed from the end of the campus that housed the library. Tom had chosen to call this number first, as it placed him within walking distance of the precious books that awaited him.

When he rang the doorbell, a wiry young man with round glasses answered

85

and held out his hand, "I'm Spike," he said.

"Tom," Tom replied as he accepted the outstretched hand that was attached to a smiling Spike. Tom was led down a dark hall that ended in three doors. Straight ahead was a bathroom, and on the left or right were two bedrooms.

"This one's yours, if you want it," Spike said, as he pushed open the door on the left. Tom looked in, there was a small bed, a desk with a lamp and a poster of the Eiffel Tower hanging on thumb tacks on one wall. Tom looked at the poster, with raised eyebrows.

"It was a gift from my friend Russ," Spike said, "You'll meet him. He's over here all the time."

"Why the picture of France?" Tom asked.

Spike laughed. "Russ is French," he said, "He and his family were refugees from the revolution, so they fled to Holland. In Holland they became missionaries for the Dutch reform church, and the church sent them to India. His mother was a surgeon, I think, and his father was an agricultural engineer." Spike fiddled with a book on the desk, and then went on.

"Russ was born and raised in Southern India. He speaks just about everything, including Hindu. He's a pretty bright guy, just watch him some day, he does crossword puzzles with a pen. Always finishes them, too." Spike stood with his arms folded across his chest.

Tom nodded, impressed. "So he's French?"

"Yeah," Spike said, "Rumor has it he was seventh in line for succession to the throne."

"Is that true?" Tom asked.

"Who knows?" Spike answered, "You can ask him yourself, if you like, but Russ doesn't really seem to care. They send food occasionally from Holland."

"Is he pre-med then?" Tom asked.

"No, he is more into research...like me," Spike said, then continued, "Anyway, the kitchen is downstairs. Sorry about the roaches, you had best keep everything in the refrigerator. We could call the landlord and tell him that the house needs fumigation, but then he would see the mess we have made of it and probably kick us all out."

Tom began unpacking his few belongings and arranged them in the desk drawers. Later he would go to the bookstore and find out what texts were required for his first semester classes. Unless there were used books for sale, he would probably read them at the library rather than spend his scarce money.

After the first few weeks, Tom's academics were proceeding well, with the exception that he was developing a growing distaste for psychology. Which was problematic since he majored in that field. He found that while he enjoyed literature and the various interpretations one was allowed to make on a poem, it should be obvious that science should be exact. Science and art were different. One was creative and one was meant to provide consistent, repeatable answers to questions. Psychology, he determined, used smoke and mirrors to pass itself off as science.

To him, it was a fine show, but inherently dishonest. Finding out what determined human motives and behavior was, of course, extremely interesting, but with psychologists, there was no consideration about the possibility that animal behavior could be inherited. Laboratory rats were bred in captivity, and many times the offspring of an aggressive rat exhibited similar traits as its parents. Psychologists accepted that as the conditioning of the parents. The young rats *learned* to be aggressive. Yet often, infant rats were separated from their parents at birth. So how could there be any parental influence?

The professors didn't take kindly to these observations and a growing schism developed between Tom and some of the faculty.

Spike and Russ agreed with Tom.

"It's all bullshit," Spike observed, "The only thing that keeps the field alive is the fact that there are no human studies. If humans were lab animals, then it would blow all their theories out of the water."

"That's a revolting thought," Russ said, "Are you suggesting we start experimenting on people?"

"What do you think the grad students are for?" Spike shot back.

"Not a selective breeding program!" Tom interjected, "Unless there's more going on up there than we know about."

But Spike was serious. "It's impossible, of course, so we'll never know the answers. The fact is, you can prove a lot of things with lab animals, but psychologists always think that humans are inherently different so they don't care."

Both Spike and Tom had been drifting away from the psych department and trying to attach themselves to another discipline. There was a possibility that the University would offer a new degree in Physiological Psychology. Every effort was being made by the three friends to align themselves with professors outside of traditional psychology. One such professor, in particular, caught Tom's attention.

Dr. Elizabeth Crosby ran the Neuroanatomy course in the physiology department. She was a small, frail looking woman with large glasses and owl eyes. In all, she probably weighed 85 pounds, but despite her diminutive stature, she was a giant in the field of anatomy. Her textbook, "The Comparative Anatomy of the Brain in Mammals, Including Man" had been the standard text for decades. The strong, yet compassionate, Dr. Crosby, Tom discovered, had never married. Instead she dedicated her life to research and science. There was a little known secret as well, that she would adopt an orphan girl, raise her and put her through college. She would then adopt another and repeat the process. Tom was never able to find out if one of the students at Michigan was the adopted child of Dr. Crosby or where she was in this humanitarian cycle, but having been familiar with hardships during his childhood, Tom adored her all the more for the selfless altruism.

As Tom delved into the inner workings of the brain, he grew in his passion and curiosity. It was beginning to make sense. The amygdala controlled *these* functions. The speech center was located *here*. The connective fibers that joined the two hemispheres across the commissure were greater in number in women than they were in men, and his beloved professor readily answered the questions that arose from his observations.

"Yes, Tom, that's true, there are more connections between the right and left brain in women than there are in men."

"But why?" Tom asked Dr. Crosby, "How can the *anatomy* be different in the genders?"

"Interesting question, Tom," Dr. Crosby replied, "But of course the anatomy *is* different. It's different in other organs, so why not the brain?"

Tom contemplated this for a moment, and then followed with the question that had been nagging at him for years.

"Then, if there is an *anatomical* difference in the brains, it follows that there would be a function for that difference, and as a result, women and men must utilize their brains differently, correct?"

Dr. Crosby smiled, and then said, "Surely you don't expect me to go down *that* road do you, Tom? I'm an anatomist, not a psychologist. But I will offer one observation; it does seem to me that since the right brain is more the center for emotions, and the left hemisphere is more the center for logic and calculations, it's interesting that women have been touted as having more feelings than men. Perhaps, and please don't quote me on this, emotions are as present in men as they are in women, but when a man compartmentalizes his thoughts in logic, he isn't plagued by the input of his feelings."

Dr. Crosby smiled a quick smile and walked away, leaving Tom to reflect on her comments.

Men had passion, he thought, or there would be a lot less poetry in the world. But men also seemed to have a higher capacity to kill, both animals and each other. Probably the lack of input from the emotional centers allowed for this. At the very least, there was more evidence for his growing philosophy that human behavior was linked to anatomical structures, regardless of what his psychology professors would say.

Tom, Russ and Spike studied constantly. All three of them found a home in physiology, and their combined dedications were appreciated. Much of the equipment at Michigan was antiquated and temperamental, so the few students who had the determination to make it work stood out from the others. One such device was a genuine museum piece. The contemporary standard machine used to measure nerve impulses was an electronic oscilloscope, but the physiology lab at Michigan used a "smoked drum" system.

It operated via taking a long stretch of paper and constructing a continuous roll out of it. Then the roll was dipped into shellac to make it sticky and then rolled in soot. Once this black sooty roll was placed on a rotating drum, measuring equipment could be connected, and the firing of neurons could be accurately measured.

Tom and Spike would spend hours setting it up, sometimes working late into the night. They would emerge from the lab victorious, but looking as if they had been cleaning chimneys.

Instead of taking short cuts to gain the expected results, they went to great pains to verify their research. The professors took note, and ultimately as a result, enough pressure was placed on administration to offer a new degree – one in Physiological Psychology.

Nearing graduation, it was a huge relief to Tom that his degree carried somewhat of a "respectable" title. Tom's only regret, in fact, was centered around the Neuroanatomy lab taught by his beloved Dr. Crosby. He had done the best he could, but he had struggled miserably with microanatomy. He was too ashamed to admit, especially to Dr. Crosby, that he had never seen, much less *used* a microscope prior to this course. The University of West Virginia didn't own one. As he fumbled through the lab course, he inwardly cursed the ineptness of West Virginia and the dignity it was costing him. At the end of the course, when Dr. Crosby pulled him aside, she was apologetic.

"I'm sorry Tom. You are my best student, but your lab work just isn't up to everything else. I'm going to have to give you an A minus."

Tom was delighted and could have kissed her, but he struggled to look serious and chagrined. He had escaped detection. She would never know his shame over his past.

Toms experience grew, even as an undergrad. Since many of the college units he transferred from West Virginia were not recognized by Michigan, Tom had acquired nearly twice the normal amount normally needed for graduation. His experience came in handy on occasion, since he was often called upon to help other students.

The most striking of these events occurred when Tom stopped into the men's room one time on his way to what he felt would surely be his most exciting class.

The professor, Dr. Donald Marquis, was to be teaching a course called, "The Neural Mechanisms of Behavior." Tom was especially excited since this particular professor was the author of the textbook by the same name. He had already read a good portion of the text in the library, and it appeared that Dr. Marquis actually was one of the very few scientists who explored the functions of the brain and attributed human behavior to the structures. The course was, in fact, a graduate seminar, but Tom had finagled a way into it, pulling heavily on his past studies and knowledge.

Tom made a quick trip into the men's room on his way to the class that first day and was alarmed to see Dr. Marquis leaning over a sink and splashing cold water on his face.

"Are you all right?" Tom asked.

Dr. Marquis looked up; his face was a pallid white. "Not really, no. I don't feel well," he said, and then to Tom, "You're Tom Law, aren't you?"

"Yes," Tom responded, "Is there something I can do for you?"

"Well, yes, Tom, as a matter of fact there is. Actually, I'm not sick, really. But I have to confess, I have a terrible affliction. I have a bad case of stage fright and I don't think I can teach this course."

Tom's face fell. He had been looking so forward to it and was bitterly disappointed at the thought of it being cancelled.

"What can I do?" Tom asked.

Dr. Marquis paused a moment, then reached into his briefcase and handed Tom a stack of papers and said, "You can teach it for me."

Tom started to protest, but Dr. Marquis cut him off. "I know you know the material, Tom. I've heard all about you. Here are the notes. Just read off of them and you'll do fine."

Stunned, Tom held the papers loosely in his hand and stood with his mouth open, as Dr. Marquis ran into a stall and started throwing up. Tom swallowed hard and looked at his watch. He had five minutes to make it into the lecture hall. When he walked in, he looked at the students all seated and prepared to take down every word from the maven, Dr. Marquis. Tom was disappointed as Dr. Marquis had special skills and knowledge and had mastered exactly what Tom wanted to learn.

Well, Tom thought to himself, this will surely test everyone's faith and a lot more.

Tom introduced himself, and before anyone could ask questions, he quickly began. He started reading from the notes, but soon decided that it would be best to back up and cover the background on the material. Pencils moved rapidly on papers, as the graduate students took notes furiously in an attempt to keep pace. Before Tom knew it, the hour was up, and class broke.

Tom collected his notes and left to find Russ and Spike.

"You're not going to *believe* what I have to do now," he said when he caught up with Spike, "I have to *teach* the graduate seminar on Neural Mechanisms of Behavior!"

Spike looked up with disinterest. He was eating a pizza and dropping globs of sauce on a borrowed textbook. "So?" Spike said, "Big deal. Everyone knows you love that shit."

Not having received the reaction he was after, Tom found Russ and tried again.

Russ, however, gave a similar reaction, and Tom gave it up as a waste of time. He would simply have to find a way to fit this into his schedule, and whether or not there would be any recognition, at least, he reassured himself, he would have the material down.

There's nothing like teaching something, he mused, to give you deeper appreciation.

Tom finished the course, then found and thanked Dr. Marquis for the faith he had placed in him.

Dr. Marquis placed a friendly hand on Tom's shoulder. "I should be thanking you, Tom. From the feedback I've heard, I made a wise decision." Dr. Marquis left the campus shortly after, and Tom was left to wonder if there was someone else that should have taught it, or if it was simply a matter of walking into a bathroom at the wrong time. Tom decided that it was a combination of the two and let it go at that.

As Russ, Tom and Spike prepared for their final year, it was approaching the time to apply for graduate school. There was no question they would be going. Undergraduate was just the preliminaries. The application procedure was arduous. Four qualifying exams of eight hours each had to be completed in a two-week period. Cramming for those exams, on top of the regular course load, placed tremendous pressure on the students and they complained about it. Some became despondent or apathetic. A few suffered from such deep depression that their peers worried about suicide attempts.

It concerned Tom, not for himself, but for the fact that the faculty almost relished in the suffering it caused the students. The brightest and the best were forced to live half-lives, delicately balanced between accomplishment and self-destruction.

Perhaps, Tom later reflected, it was this attitude that caused him to take action against the faculty.

A petition was drafted. It stated that the students would discontinue attendance of all courses, including lab and research projects, unless the four qualifying exams were split. Two exams should be given in the fall months, and the final two in the spring.

The faculty scoffed at the petition and ignored it. Tom rallied the students into a protest, complete with picket signs. Some of the students were volunteers from other disciplines, and in fact had nothing to gain or lose by the protest; rather, they were the type that simply enjoyed rebellion. But many were scientists like Tom. They wanted resolution, and their nerves had been stretched to the point of breaking. The diversion created a sense of control and relief.

Tom was called into the Dean's office.

"Mr. Law," The Dean said with a mixture of condescension and reproof, "I have been made aware of the fact that you do not think you can pass the entrance exams for graduate school. For years our graduate students, the very ones who now hold doctorates and are viable members of the scientific community, have been able to accomplish what you find to be too demanding."

Tom fought back his anger and responded coolly, "I'm just another student," he said, "and as a representative of the student body protesting the exam structure, I would like to point out that the ultimate purpose for our being here is to learn." Tom switched from one foot to his other, then continued. "The exams require massive amounts of studying. To place all four of them in a two-week period precludes our ability to focus on the courses we're attending, and that reduces the quality of our course work and the information we garner from those classes. As a University that wants its students to walk away from here with a high level of training, this should be a matter of importance to you."

The Dean was visibly irritated and responded, "Are you saying that the students we have graduated before are lacking in knowledge?"

"What I'm saying is," Tom responded, "That it's very simple. Students will cram for any exam you give them. They'll do whatever is necessary. But there's always a price to pay when expectations are unreasonable. If you insist on keeping the entrance exams as scheduled, then your top students, myself included, will discontinue our research. We'll have to stop teaching in your labs, and your faculty will have to take more time out from their grant proposals, and this will impact the University funding."

The Dean was furious at the blatant disregard for his authority. Who did this *child* think he was? He belonged on a political campus, one that fostered left-wing liberals, not Michigan. Yet, the threats of a full force student strike did not set well. There was truth to the fact that much of the funding that kept this expensive University running came from research grants. Alumni contributions were down. The economy impacted everything, and the dean was constantly walking a tight rope keeping the whole mess from collapsing. After contemplating for a moment, the dean said, "I think you're out of bounds, Tom, but if you find that our exam structure is beyond your capabilities, in spite of the fact that throughout history others have been up to our standards, then I will consider your proposal."

Tom chaffed at the dig. The Dean knew this was not about him, but the issue was being made personal.

"Thanks," said Tom, and he turned on his heel and walked out.

One week later the administration made an announcement. Qualifying exams for graduate school were to be taken five months apart, two in the fall and two in the spring. The faculty was quick to point out that the concession was not in response to the student strike; rather it was a scheduling dilemma for the exam proctors and spreading the exams out gave them time to attend to their busy schedules.

One hour after the announcement was made, Tom was waiting outside the Deans office. When he was admitted, the Dean looked wearily up and said, "What is it now, Tom, another ultimatum?"

"I'm ready for the exams," Tom said, "I want to take them now."

"I beg your pardon?" the Dean said.

"This week. I'm ready. I want to take all four exams." Tom said flatly.

The Dean's face flushed. "Fine," he said.

For thirty-two hours Tom sat alone in a small room. His only interruption was when a proctor walked into the room, looked suspiciously around and walked out again, closing the door behind him. There were hundreds of questions. The ones on neuroanatomy and physiology were simple; Tom could have passed them a year ago without much effort. Biochemistry was easy, there was only one right answer, and that was simply a matter of applying the right formula and completing the calculation.

Psychology gave him some trouble. He just didn't care enough about it to dedicate his mind to finding the answer they wanted. He found himself sidetracked with rebuttals to the postulates. In his mind's eye, he debated the "correct" answer with alternate conclusions. This cost him time, but he gripped himself to play the game and answer the questions with a guilty infraction on his personal ethics. On the fourth day he handed in the final exam to the proctor and walked home.

Spike was waiting for him. "How did it go?" Spike asked anxiously.

"Fine," Tom replied, "When you take it, you'll pass...no problem."

"I'm not taking them all at once like you just did," Spike said, "That's just crazy. What are you trying to prove anyway? You led this strike and won...so why the blatant slap in the face to the administration?"

Tom was tired and sat down heavily. He accepted the beer that Spike offered him.

"I guess..." he began, "I guess I just have a problem with authority. Probably, if I stopped to think about it, I'm angry with the domineering and senseless oppression of my father."

"Ah," Spike said, "The 'ol Oedipus complex...yes...that's going around."

Tom smiled. "No intentions of marrying my mother, but...killing my father? That doesn't seem too far fetched at this moment. I guess petty officialdom flaunting its authority with no concern for an individual's feelings hits close to home. I hate it. I don't respect the office. Either the man is worthy or he isn't. End of story."

"Take a break," Spike said, "We are all off to grad school soon, and it'll be different there. No longer the slaves of tenured professors. Instead we'll be working towards our own personal fame and fortunes."

"I hope so," Tom finished.

Tom received his scores one week later. He passed with "highest honors" in all four exams. It surprised even Tom, since he was certain that the questions in psychology would undermine him. Yet, he had made the decision to answer the questions with what the examiners had wanted, not with what he felt to be true. It sickened him in a way, but he felt he could claim a high moral ground on the victory over the system, by forcing the faculty to offer the exams spread out and then taking them all in a single week.

That had never been done before at Michigan. It was unheard of. There were repercussions in the administration and Tom was ever more the pariah, yet there was little they could do about it. Highest honors and his 4.0 GPA made it impossible for them to not admit him to the graduate program.

As far as the graduate program was concerned, he had to consider the playing field. Dr. Pierson, the professor who advocated Gestalt psychology hated Tom and the feeling was mutual. He would be someone to steer clear of in the future if at all possible.

Dr. Blackwell was clueless, but he had a ton of research money that he somehow garnered from the US military. Dr. Blackwell was not hostile towards Tom, and he did have funds, so possibly it would be advantageous to culture a relationship there. Tom's mind was calculating all the avenues he could take to leverage his situation. It was politics, pure and simple, and nothing more. Research could be done and would be done, but the key to success was not the help he would receive, rather it was in avoiding the obstacles of obstructionists. Petty jealously played a major roll in the university, and Tom had already made a host of enemies. He would have to watch his step in the years that lay ahead.

Graduate school passed quickly for Tom and his friends. He immediately learned that if you don't get in the way of the professors, they won't make a point of harassing you. Most of all he learned the power of results. Professors were under constant pressure to publish research papers, and regardless of their past successes, each new semester the slate was wiped clean and they were required to start anew. The graduate students who contributed to research were highly sought after by the faculty. It became immediately known who was brilliant and who was not.

Tom, Spike and Russ were among the top producers and their abilities were well known. Their rebellious attitudes were tolerated since their value was so great. Yet in spite of their brilliance, the faculty had many ways to keep the three under a degree of control.

There was always the leverage of the Doctorate degree to use against them. Their future careers depended on it, and regardless of their brilliance, they could not progress far in the world of science without credentials.

Eventually they came to an impasse over the required courses in Personality Theory. Tom and his friends were accustomed to the physiology departments' manner of testing theories. A hypothesis about behavior was tested and the results were documented. Anyone who challenged the results could repeat the test and either gain the same results or refute them. The courses on personality theory were based on sociological observations alone, and the professors would launch into dissertations on behavior models, using examples derived from human observations, and the students were expected to accept it as gospel.

Tom, Spike and Russ refused to take the courses, and the administration calmly informed them that they would not receive degrees unless they did. Finally relenting, the students sat for the course, but they made it a point to harass the instructor. Challenging to the point of belligerence, Tom and friends made sure the professor was just as miserable as they were. Exams were multiple choice, so the professor could not fail them, although he desperately wanted to. At the end of the semester they all received highest marks.

"What a waste of time," Russ said, "Thank God that's over."

"I won't do it again," Spike said with finality.

Spikes resolve was put to the test the very next semester. Dr. Blackie, the famed psychologist who devised the "Blackie test", a personality determinant that centered on a small black dog, was teaching a course on psychology. During the first day of the semester, Dr. Blackie began his lecture by reading, verbatim, from his book. The students had already purchased the book, as it was required reading, and as Dr. Blackie turned to the fourth page and continued reading in a sonorous monotone, Spike leapt up from his chair, flung the book on the floor and exclaimed, "This is bullshit!" and stormed out of the lecture hall.

After an embarrassed silence, the professor continued where he had left off, and Tom and Russ sighed and returned their attention to daydreaming about physiology lab experiments. Tom glanced at Russ, who wore a small smile. They knew that Spike was the one with enough personal integrity to protest, but they also knew that he would not receive a degree unless he returned and apologized.

As it turned out, Spike would not return. The administration made it very clear that he would not be graduating, not just from this incident alone, but also for the fact that Spike had also refused to take the required foreign language.

"I'm not taking French!" Spike had told the faculty, "French…what the hell does that have to do with my research?" he had exclaimed.

Spike had a just argument, since he had recently published, "The Theory Of Visual Detection" which was extremely popular in the scientific community and it was revolutionizing the field of Psychophysics.

"They can have their damn degree," Spike said, "I don't need it."

Nearing graduation, Tom was concerned for Spike. "Yes, I know it is all bullshit," Tom admitted, "But it would be easy for you to pass these filler courses…why not just play the game and get your degree?"

"Tom," Spike responded, "You of all people know that the brain isn't a black box whose inner workings are irrelevant to behavior. You've been in the labs for years now. You know the effects of neurotransmitters on the brain and how the delicate balances radically change an animal's actions. How can you even listen to the theories that anatomical structures are irrelevant? Even as an undergrad, you were questioning the connective fibers between the two halves of the brain and how women have more of them." Spike was standing on one foot and then the other as he continued.

"You yourself suggested that the anatomical differences could be responsible for behavior differences. Yet, if you try to discuss this with psychologists, you're slapped down. They don't want to hear it, yet the solid evidence stares them in the face. How can you reconcile this with what you know?"

Spike was striking at a soft spot for Tom.

It irritated Tom that he had to swallow his pride. It also irritated him that Spike had enough defiance to spit in the face of the administration. Yet Spike could afford it, and Tom could not. Spike's family had enough money to support him, and even without a degree, he would not find it difficult to survive. Tom couldn't share this information with Spike, and certainly not with Russ, who seemed to suffer from an endless flow of cash, but Tom was on his own. His family lived in a constant state of semi-starvation, and they were completely out of the picture as far as any help was concerned.

His father would probably be happy if he failed, and his suggestion would be to return to the farm where he belonged and lend a hand with the endless physical labor.

Tom was running out of tuition money and becoming desperate. He had filed applications for a fellowship, and with his academic excellence, there was absolutely no reason for him not to receive it. Yet the toes he had treaded so heavily upon in the past were still smarting. The administration relished in denying him any help. With only two semesters remaining, Tom faced the possibility of having to drop out.

It was Dr. Blackwell who eventually came to Tom's aid. Dr. Blackwell was still sitting on a pile of military funding. It was a mystery how he had achieved it, especially in light of the fact that he didn't seem to know what to do with it. Any budget money left unspent was cut the following year, so Dr. Blackwell kept himself busy purchasing state of the art equipment and trying to look busy. Tom felt he was worthless as a researcher, but at least he didn't hold any grudges against Tom and his friends.

Possibly, Tom conjectured, there was jealously amongst the faculty at the providence Dr. Blackwell found, and as such, he was as much an outcast as Tom.

As Tom entered the lab, Dr. Blackwell glanced up in surprise. He had been fiddling with a new piece of equipment, a stereotactic probe, by the looks of it. It was apparent he didn't have a feel for how the device was meant to work.

"Why, hello, Mr. Law," Dr. Blackwell said, "I hope you came here to help me with this contraption." Tom smiled amiably. For all his other faults, Dr. Blackwell was not egotistical.

"The truth is, I came to ask you for a favor."

"Oh? Tell me."

Tom regarded the lab bench for a moment, his mind flashed to the lifetime of poverty he had endured and pride must once again be swallowed in order to move ahead.

"I can't pay tuition next semester," Tom said.

"Ah, I see. Well, why don't you apply for a Fellowship? I know the University has the funds, and your record stands on its own."

"I did," Tom said, "It was denied."

Dr. Blackwell sighed. "I see. You probably don't have many friends in administration…I know how that is."

By now Tom had moved up to the probe guide and was assembling it to fit the filament. Dr. Blackwell watched as Tom placed the device over the top of a round piece of modeling clay. Then he guided the probe gently into the clay. His movements were reduced mechanically so that the probe could be gently inserted with great accuracy.

Dr. Blackwell watched with interest. "I have an idea," he said, "You can come to work for me. If you help with my research projects, I'll see to it you graduate."

Tom looked up with a smile of relief. While Dr. Blackwell may not be the brightest of all researchers, he was a decent man, and for once, Tom felt that someone was actually willing to lend a helping hand.

"Thank you. Thank you very much, you don't know how much this means to me."

"Can you give me four hours a day?" Dr. Blackwell asked.

"I can give you seven," Tom replied, and with that, his crisis was over.

Tom graduated with highest honors, again, that spring, and in the interim, he advanced Dr. Blackwell's project by at least a year.

He said goodbye to his few friends, including Dr. Blackwell and prepared for his attendance in the post doctorate program at Johns Hopkins.

Russ had also graduated with high honors and had been offered a Fullbright scholarship overseas.

Spike Tanner did not graduate. Instead he left with a certificate from Michigan that stated he had completed all requirements, minus French. He was hired by a biomedical research institute and displayed the certificate with pride, amongst his various commendations for research, on his office wall.

When Tom arrived at Johns Hopkins, it was like coming home. Or maybe, he thought, this is what heaven is like, you see everyone you respect and admire, and they are waiting for you with open arms. Instead of petty jealousy, there was work, earnest, exciting work, from which flowed publication after publication. Ensconced in his own private lab, Tom was left alone to explore and indulge his curiosity. It was a shock at first, and it took a while for Tom to stop glancing nervously over his shoulder, expecting a faculty member to walk in the door and demand explanations for the time spent. Instead, the faculty was there to offer guidance, if needed.

Tom had a doctorate now, and it was assumed that he knew what to do with it. At first, Tom dove into visual research projects. He had enough ideas on the current theories to conduct some simple experiments that should be easy to publish. Still nervous about proving himself, he published several research articles in rapid succession on the optic nerve, and while there were no accolades from administration, there was also no indication that they were particularly concerned with Tom's efforts.

Tom began to feel confident, and his interests returned to human behavior. There were so many questions, and all the answers he had been given were suspect. For once, he could begin to seek some of the answers without censorship.

A probe had to be made. The brain was the most delicate of all tissues and to delve deeply into it, one must have a probe that was no larger than a fifteenth of the size of a human hair. Anything larger and it destroyed the tissues as it penetrated, rendering any results useless. Hundreds of attempts had been made; several of the top scientists in the world had constructed probes made of everything from tungsten to silver or gold.

All of them were either thin enough to not cause damage, yet too flexible to make it to the deeper tissues, or they were thick enough to resist bending, but damaged the tissue they penetrated. Thousands upon thousands of dollars had been spent, but to no avail.

Tom was determined to find the answer. The mapping of the brain was under way, but so far, only the outer structures had been explored. If he could find a way to make it inside, he had a chance to find the untold secrets. He might even have a chance to find out what motivated animals in every potential situation. In particular, he wondered about reproductive behavior.

There was a nagging thought in the back of his mind. He had studied human evolution and was intimate with the theories. He knew that if an organism did not reproduce, it did not exist as a species in the next generation. It could go hungry, it could be too cold or too hot, but those conditions did not have the same ultimate impact on the future. Everything centered on reproduction. For bacteria, it was simple. Divide as often as you can. That was a simple matter of acquiring enough food to replicate. But higher organisms, there was more investment there. On the one hand, lobsters had a good technique. They would deposit three thousand eggs and let fate take them where it would. Some would survive, most would not, but the investment of the lobster was minimal. It was one way to go.

Humans and more complex animals had a different strategy.

Only a precious few offspring would be made, and those few would take years upon years of nurturing to reach reproductive age. It seemed to Tom, that the most obvious difference in these tactics was the brain. A lobster had just as efficient a spinal column as a human, but like the rest of the more simple animals, the smaller the brain, the less investment in nurturing the young. There had to be a connection, Tom surmised, and the secret lay in the inner structures of the brain. A probe had to be constructed that would go deep.

Over a pitcher of beer, Tom offered his theories to Kiefer Hartline. Kiefer occupied the lab directly below Tom and was constantly helping Tom solve some of his laboratory dilemmas.

Kiefer had been working on optical stimulations and had made the discovery that there were ways to sequence light images in primitive eyes, such as the eyes of horseshoe crabs, which inhibited certain photoreceptors. From that, he had extrapolated how the crab uses his eye in horizon detection. It was brilliant research and eloquently done, and as such, there were rumors that Keifer would possibly win the Nobel Prize.

Tom drew heavily on Kiefer's knowledge. On one occasion, Tom had needed to build a shielded cage, one that could measure minute electrical impulses across a nerve, without interference from the radio waves transmitted twenty-four hours a day from the local radio stations.

"That's easy," Kiefer said, "Just build a Faraday cage."

"I know *that*, Kiefer," Tom said, "But I don't have the budget. A Faraday cage costs thousands of dollars in copper wire. I just don't have it."

"Well…." Kiefer said as he contemplated, "Do this then. Take a cardboard box, one about the size of what they sell feminine hygiene products in and line it with aluminum foil. I think that would work."

Tom appreciated the irony, as the experiment involved reproductive habits in lab rats.

"OK, I'll try it."

Later Tom found that while the Kotex box he had stolen from his wife was the right size and shape, the shielding needed to be grounded, and the lab lacked a sufficient means of isolating the metal conductors. Kiefer was again called into service. Pounding down the steps to the lab below, Tom burst in on Kiefer.

"I need to ground it," he said flatly. Kiefer looked up from his work,

"OK, do this. Wait until dark tonight and dig a hole in the dirt outside the lab. Fill it with charcoal that you have soaked in salt water and place a copper plate in the middle of it. When you run a wire up to your window and connect it, you should have adequate grounding."

"Thanks," Tom said, and bounded back up the stairs.

All of Kiefer's ideas had worked so far, so Tom once again sat with him in hopes that they could come up with a solution.

"A probe," Kiefer said, "I see the problem. You need something small and rigid, that conducts electricity so you can measure the activity of the brain cells right?"

"Yes," Tom said, "and everything they have tried so far has failed."

"Everything?" Kiefer said.

"Everything. Including metal filaments that cost thousands to make. The thin ones can't be guided. They're too flexible."

"Have you considered modifying the stereo tactic device so it can guide them?"

"Yes, I have," Tom said, "I have a new design that I should probably patent. It's superior to anything out there, but still it won't prevent the probes from going wherever they choose."

Kiefer looked interested. "About that device, why not patent it? You could make some money."

"No time," Tom said, "I would rather get the right probe and get on with it. Besides, anything I invent here at Hopkins belongs to the university. I would only be making them money and I don't care about that. I want the probe."

Kiefer stared into his beer. "I give up," he said, "I can't think of anything conductive that's rigid enough when it has the small diameter that you need. Sorry."

Tom sat for a moment in dismay. The great Kiefer had always provided ready solutions to Tom's problems, but it was unreasonable to expect him to have every answer. As Tom stared into his own mug, he thought about the alcohol lamps he had used to melt glass.

In his undergraduate career, there were experiments on sea urchin eggs that involved glass pipettes. Sea Urchin eggs were wonderful for the fact that they were huge, and even the most bumbling of students could find them and fertilize them with a glass pipette. As a side benefit, the university didn't look objectionably when it came to the reproductive studies of sea urchins. Take a swab on the vagina of a female rat and it caused raised eyebrows amongst administration, but they could fertilize sea urchins all day with impunity.

"Have you made glass pipettes before?" Tom asked Kiefer.

"Sure," Kiefer said, "Heat up a hollow glass tube, pull it rapidly apart and viola! You have a pipette!"

"How thin do you think you could make one?" Tom asked.

"Pretty thin, I think," Kiefer said, "But even if you can get down to a few microns, you still have a nonconductive material, so what's the use?"

"I have an idea," Tom said.

That night, Kiefer and Tom heated and pulled over thirty pieces of glass until they had one that was the right diameter. It was a simple and primitive technique they used. Several alcohol burners were placed in a row and a glass tube was gently heated over the flames. Kiefer stood on one end, and Tom stood on the other, ready to pull the glass rapidly apart when the temperature was just right. If they pulled too soon, the glass would break. If too late, it would sag and bend, and they would have to start over.

Finally, they had a tube that looked right. They gently laid it on the lab bench and looked it over under magnification.

"I don't see any holes," Kiefer said, "This might be the one, but I still don't know how to make it conduct electricity. You can't measure the electrical currents of brain cells unless your probe is conductive."

"Of course not, Kiefer," Tom said, "We have to fill it with a conductor, like sodium chloride."

Kiefer looked perplexed, then brightened. "I've got it!" he said, "I'll set up a vacuum on one end of the tube to pull in the solution!"

"Won't work," Tom said, "The glass is too fragile. Besides, I have a better idea. I'll soak the tube in a high concentration of potassium chloride over night, and then change the solution to sodium chloride. By morning it should be ready."

"How's that solution going to fill the inside of the tube?" Kiefer asked.

"The same way water gets from the roots of trees to the leaves. There's no pump, it's all capillary action. By morning, we'll have a conductive probe that I can use." Tom was smiling now.

Kiefer left the lab, and Tom placed the filament of glass into a vat of electrolyte. The thin part of the tube disappeared from view as he submerged it, and all that was visible was the thick portion of glass that had not melted in the flame and been stretched to microscopic dimension.

Tom made his bed on a small cot that had become his perennial home.

Two hours later he got up and examined the tube under a microscope. The dyed solution had filled it, and he exchanged the tube into another container that had surgical saline solution in it. The ions would exchange, and the probe would be ready soon.

Tom collapsed again on the cot, and wondered if he should have called his wife. She knew where he was, of course, but she never called him at the lab. Tom tended to be short with her when he was working, and yet he was always working. He quickly forgot about it and his mind drifted off. He awoke two hours later. The sky was beginning to lighten, and Tom groggily checked the probe. Under a microscope, he discovered a perfectly filled tube. "Bless those trees," he said to himself. It had worked.

The new probe was placed into immediate use, along with the modified stereo tactic guide. Researchers were skeptical at first, but when the probe made it to the center of the brain without breaking or bending, the surgery room became jubilant. Tom and Kiefer observed as the probe approached the amygdala, a deep tissue that had never been explored before. An oscilloscope registered electrical changes at the tip of the probe, and nearing its destination there was a steady rhythm across the screen.

"What's that?" Kiefer asked.

"A single neuron firing," Tom said, "Its stopped just outside a single cell, and that's its base rhythm."

There were raised eyebrows as the surgery continued. Neurosurgery was an infant science. Physicians throughout the world needed to know the damages that would be caused if certain structures were sacrificed in attempts to remove cancerous tumors.

Pharmaceutical treatments of severe diseases depended on finding the effects of drugs on the various tissues, and thus far, only the outer reaches of the brain had been accessible. It was the beginning of a new era. Tom's probe had been the breakthrough they needed.

That night a group from the university were informally assembled at the local pub. Tom sat next to Bill McElroy, the famous biochemist whose class Tom had just recently taken. Bill had won the Nobel Prize for discovering the enzymes that fireflies use to light their bodies. It had been a masterpiece of elegance in chemistry, and the potential applications of the enzymes were keeping engineers up late at night. Bill had a sense of humor, and he had named the paired enzymes "Luciferin and Luciferase". Tom had commented on the names and asked Bill about their significance.

"Hell fire," Bill replied, "You know, Lucifer – the Devil. I had a devil of a time isolating those enzymes, so it seemed appropriate. By the way, nice work on the probe, Tom."

"Thanks," Tom said, "They'll come up with something better soon, but this gets us started anyway." Tom was weary, but smiling. His favorite people were sitting near him, and each of them was either famous or soon to be.

Kiefer sat across the table near Dr. Hamberger. They were having a discussion about the surgical unit Dr. Hamberger had invented. Tom had worked with Dr. Hamberger, and he knew the challenges associated with the surgery unit.

Instead of a scalpel, the "knife" was a thin electric probe that cauterized the tissue as it cut through it. The supreme advantage this had was that it controlled the bleeding, making the surgical area easier to see. The problem Dr. Hamberger was experiencing was that the electrical resistance of the cauterized tissue changed, and as a result the device would not cut – or worse, if the current was turned up to compensate, the tissue became too hot and caused excessive damage.

Tom caught a part of the conversation.

"...why not have Tom here take a look at it. I've seen some of his lab equipment, he's good with electronics," Kiefer was saying.

Dr. Hamberger looked over at Tom, who was looking as if he had not slept in days. "Want to take a look at it, Tom?" he asked.

"Glad to," Tom replied. He wanted nothing more than to continue with his brain research, yet one did not turn down an invitation to help.

The next morning Tom reported to Dr. Hamberger's office. The scientist was out, but Tom took one of the experimental surgical units back to his lab and began his dissection of it. His mind was preoccupied with the probe and the secrets it would uncover, but the diversion of some electronic circuitry in all its comparative simplicity relative to the brain was an antidote to his racing mind. The circuit needed something to tell it how much power to use. A surgeon could not have the sensitivity to know, and after a few days of experimentation, Tom had the machine working.

Dr. Hamberger had left Tom alone, and Tom took it upon himself to send his modifications out for publication in a scientific journal. When the fully operational device was returned to Dr. Hamberger's office, Tom found two other faculty members in the lab. They were discussing something about grant applications, but abruptly stopped as Tom walked in.

"Done," Tom said, as he placed the unit on the counter, "It works now. Perfectly."

The scientists approached the machine and one asked Tom, "What did you do to it?"

Tom removed the cover and exposed the circuits. "Here, this regulates the voltage." Tom was indicating a new addition to the machine, and the component was unique in design.

Dr. Hamberger laughed. "This could be patented!" he exclaimed.

"I know," Tom said, "I just filed an application." There was stunned silence, and then Dr. Hamberger regarded Tom with a different look.

"You realize, Tom, that anything you patent while attending Johns Hopkins belongs to the university."

Tom looked at the three men; "I published my results last week," he said. "It's already out there."

Dr. Hamberger stared back, then gave a short laugh and clapped a friendly hand on Tom's shoulder. The other two men were smiling, and Dr. Hamberger chuckled and said, "Good for you, Tom. Good for you." And he then returned to his discussion with the others.

Tom left and considered what had just taken place. Normally his defiance initiated a power struggle that usually ended with attempts at petty revenge. But Johns Hopkins was different. These great men respected one another and loved science. It was the love of advancing the research that they held above all else, and Tom was doing his part. Tom smiled as he walked back to his lab. He was anxious to return to his own work. Anxious to continue his contributions, and now, more than ever, he felt free to be himself.

Experiments with Tom's probe advanced at a rapid rate. Already the amygdala had been mapped, and a famous experiment was being popularized in the media. The location in the brain that allowed for rage had been discovered, and when a microscopic lesion was introduced there, any animal, including predators, became completely docile. Tom found it all very interesting, but still there was no indication of the truth of his theory – the thought that the brain in some way controlled reproductive behavior.

It was within a few days of Tom's reflections when Kiefer stepped into Tom's lab and said, "Tom, you had better come and take a look at this."

"What is it?" Tom asked.

"They set a probe into the Hypothalamus of a female rat, and she's acting very strange." Tom followed Keifer to a surgical lab and walked up to the enclosure. The rat seemed healthy and normal in every respect, except for the top of her small skull, which was lacking hair and had a healing scar running along the line of the surgical entry point.

"Where did you create the lesion?" Tom asked.

Evan, the researcher answered, "Anterior hypothalamus. It's very small, just a few cells wide."

"What is it she's doing differently?" Tom asked, his curiosity peaked.

"It's a matter of what she is not doing," Evan answered, "She refuses to have anything to do with male rats, but in all other respects she appears normal."

Tom examined the rat carefully. To all intents and purposes she seemed unharmed. He reflected a moment on the plight of rats as experimental animals. It seemed a cruel twist of fate that they were subjected to experimentation, and yet, the sacrifices they inadvertently made were the foundation of modern medicine. It was easy for animal rights activists to protest against the studies, yet take any fifty of the activists and you would find a good portion of them utilizing insulin, pain relievers or a host of other medical products and procedures that came about solely as a result of animal research. It was easy, Tom thought, to sit in a restaurant eating a steak when you were not the one who had to kill the cow.

Nevertheless, Tom and all others he knew of took great pains to use compassion in their surgeries. Anesthetics were used liberally, and the animals, even rats, were well cared for.

This female was healthy. One animal Tom knew by now was rats, and the young female he held in his hand sniffed energetically and tried to climb out of his hands. Tom gently placed her in a cage with a male, who approached her and attempted to sniff.

She jerked and bit at the male, who quickly retreated.

"Let me see something here," Tom said. He took a swab and gently took a smear of the female's vagina. He then prepared a microscope slide and examined the cells under high power.

"It's cornified," Tom said, "She's not in estrous. That's why she wants nothing to do with males."

"But she *has* to be!" Evan exclaimed, "This should be the *middle* of her cycle."

"Well then, something's amiss," Tom said, "I'll prepare an injection of estrogen. We'll get her back on cycle and see what happens."

Tom administered the hormones that would make the female reproductively fertile and receptive to mating. After waiting the appropriate time, she was reintroduced to the male rat, yet while she was biologically receptive, her attitude was unchanged. She would have nothing to do with the male.

Tom was careful. This was exactly the information he had been searching for, yet he could not allow his excitement get the best of him. It would be too easy to miss something in his exuberance. Years ago, an infamous experiment had been conducted. A researcher had determined that a flatworm could learn to run a maze. When the brain tissue of the worm was fed to a new flatworm, the new one could run the maze, just as if it retained the information of its predecessor. The experiment had been repeated over and over with similar results. A theory was being developed that ingested brain tissue carried information within it that could be assimilated, and it took a long while before the discovery was made that subtle nuances in the way the experiment was set up had skewed the results. Flatworms, it turned out, do not learn by ingesting brain tissue nor do any other animals. Yet the lesson was there, a scientist's first responsibility is to disprove what they believe to be true. That way, there would be no errors or misconceptions.

Tom set out fervently to disprove his theory that the hypothalamus was the key to reproduction. Dozens of experiments were conducted, yet ultimately Tom could not disprove his theories. The brain was in control of mating desire, and the hypothalamus was the structure responsible. It was interesting, Tom thought, how close in proximity the hypothalamus was to the pituitary gland. A multitude of secretions were known to originate in the pituitary, many of which controlled such things as lactation in pregnant women. He wondered that if, in time, there would be a connection discovered.

Tom realized that he was on the cusp of exciting discoveries, and he had trouble sleeping at night. His dreams carried vivid displays of complex molecules and enzymes. Sometimes they would join and change shape. Occasionally he would wake with a start and attempt to remember what he has seen in the dream, but usually it faded faster than he could get to a pen and pad and make notes. Even when he did scratch out ideas, he found them enigmatic in the morning when he was fully awake. He stuffed the scraps of paper into an envelope and shoved it into a drawer.

Maybe, some day, he would go back over the hieroglyphics and try to make sense of them.

Tom was close to graduation from Hopkins, but he thought little of it. His daily routine had kept him so preoccupied that the months passed seamlessly. There were few things to punctuate the changes in the days of the week or even the weekends for that matter.

Tom had been in communication with his family, but only superficially, until he had a call from his mother. She called one day and in a shaky voice told Tom that his father was dying. He had suffered another heart attack, and the doctors didn't think he would survive another one. Tom calmed her down, and then asked to speak to his father.

A tired voice came on the phone. "Hello, Tom," the voice said, "I'm dying."

"Hello, dad," Tom said, "Yes, so I hear. But I have a proposition for you. I'm on the faculty here at Hopkins, and I think we can save you with an experimental surgery."

"Are *you* going to do the surgery?" the voice said with some derision.

Tom quelled his irritation, and then said, "No, dad, I'm not. But I'll assist. It's experimental, as I said, but I think it'll work."

"What have you been doing there all this time?" Tom's father asked.

"Brain research," Tom replied. "And some other things," he added.

"So, you think you know anything about my heart?" Toms father said, then before Tom could answer, "You realize that all the men in our family die young of heart attacks. No sense in denying it. Your grandpa died at 52, and I am going to die just like him."

"Come out, dad," Tom pleaded, "If you die on the operating table, then you die. But at least you'll have given it a shot."

There was a long pause, and then the voice said, "If I come out and do this, what will be the side effects?"

Tom thought for a moment. It was true that what he was considering would have side effects. In fact, if they successfully completed the bilateral sympathectomy, as Tom was going to propose, then his father would be forever impotent. But, Tom thought, he would be alive, and while it might not do much to improve his fathers' disposition, it would, by and large, be a good thing for his mother.

"No important side effects," Tom said.

"OK," his father said, and then hung up the phone.

The next week Tom directed the surgery. It was successful, and his fathers' life was saved. Several months later the elder Mr. Law called Tom and started berating,

"What the hell, Tom! I can't get an erection!"

"Yes, well," Tom said, "There is a new development in this procedure. It seems that your condition is permanent and there is nothing I can do about it."

"But…" his father started, then Tom cut him off.

"How is your heart, dad?"

"My *heart* is fine, Tom, but dammit!"

"I know," Tom said, "and I sympathize, but at least you'll live, probably another twenty years or more, so you can still help mom around the house."

"Tom, you did this…" but Tom hung the phone up before his father could finish. He had not been speaking that much with his father anyway, he mused, so this would not make matters all that much worse.

Later, he was to find his father indeed lived to be seventy-two, setting a new family record, but true to his nature, his father never fully forgave Tom. Perhaps he was right, Tom thought, it came down to a matter of values.

Tom finished his post doctorate tenure at Johns Hopkins abruptly. It was as if he had suddenly left his family and the door was shut behind him and the locks were changed. Kiefer had already left and said goodbye, and there were farewells from the permanent faculty, but there was little fanfare. He was done there, and once again he had no idea where to go or what to do with his life. So caught up in research, he had been, that he had spent absolutely no time planning his next steps. It was unlike him, but he reflected, it was a result of the fact that he had been enjoying life too much to think of anything else. He had lost weight. He often forgot to eat. He suspected his marriage was in shambles, but could not be sure. Long ago, the wife he married while in graduate school at Michigan had learned that Tom was devoted solely to his research. He felt he hardly knew the woman he called his wife, and sometimes when he introduced her at a cocktail party, he stammered when he said her name. He knew the names of thousands of anatomical structures, but a living, breathing person that was the mother of his children was more a stranger than certain species of bacteria. Serattia Marcessans left a unique red mark in its colonies on petri dishes, but his wife did not seem to leave any distinguishing marks at all. She was just there.

Tom realized he was neglecting her. Yet try as he might, he could not pull himself away from research. He was not sure what kept the marriage together, and with a guilty realization, he discovered that he did not particularly care. He was discovering the secrets of the brain – the mind. That was more important than anything.

Still, there would now be bills to pay and the details of their mundane life faced him. He needed work, and most importantly, he needed to find a way to continue his research.

On a whim, Tom picked up a phone and called Dr. Blackwell at Michigan. Dr. Blackwell was out of his office, but he returned the call on the next day.

"Tom! How was Johns Hopkins?" he asked.

"Great," Tom said, "Really great. I have some ideas."

"Bring them over," Richard said, "I'm still working on visual detection and the Navy wants some results soon."

Tom smiled to himself. The military was still pouring money in the direction of Richard Blackwell, and still he had not produced the results they were after. This would be perfect. He could advance the project in a minimal amount of time, and siphon off some of the money to be used in other areas.

"I'll be there Monday," Tom said, and Dr. Blackwell told him to find a lab when he arrived and to get started.

Chapter Seven

...hear the great teeth gnash
and rush across the table to the edge...

When Tom arrived back at the University of Michigan, he had mixed emotions. This was where he had begun, and it should seem familiar, yet everything was foreign to him. He was not a student any longer, he was an employee, and the political machinery that had controlled him before was still focused on the students. In fact, no one even seemed to know he was there.

He decided to stop by the Dean's office and make mention of the fact he was back, then thought better of it. What purpose could it serve, the Dean probably hated Tom, and the feeling was mutual. Better, he thought, to stay low and remain anonymous.

Dr. Blackwell was gone for the entire week, Tom discovered upon his arrival, and there were no messages left as to where Tom was to begin. In fact, the secretary had no idea that Tom had been hired, and seemed irritated that Tom was trying to find office space.

"Dr. Blackwell will be back in a week," the secretary said with a dismissive tone, "and you can check with him then."

"In a pig's eye," Tom murmured under his breath, and he left the office.

As Tom wandered aimlessly about the campus, in a light drizzle that had just begun to fall, he noticed a new building. It was three stories tall and placed close to the medical center. The building was barely completed, as there was scaffolding still in place on the western edifice. Painter's supplies had been left hanging on ropes, and Tom surmised that the rain had interrupted their work for the day. He tried the front door and found it open. Inside were office spaces with labs adjacent; probably this was to be a research facility for the medical students.

Instead of climbing the stairs, Tom went down. There was a basement with primitive partitions, yet electrical outlets and plumbing had been stubbed every ten feet. The area might be slated for storage, with the potential for later improvements that would allow for the expansion of the research center. Tom set his pack down on the dusty counter, and reaching inside, pulled out his name placard. Dr. O. Thomas Law, it said. He had removed it from the front of his office at Johns Hopkins on his way out. The back was still sticky, and he pressed it on the wall next to the door into the largest room. When he found a phone, he called maintenance and was eventually connected with the supervisor.

"This is Dr. Law," Tom said, "When will my office be completed? I'm here and I only have a few days to produce results or Dr. Blackwell will have my hide."

"I'm sorry?" the voice on the other end said, "Who is this?"

"Law," Tom replied. "Dr. Law. I'm in my office, and it's not completed. In fact, none of the equipment I ordered is here. The Navy's waiting. How am I supposed to get anything done without the equipment?" Tom demanded.

There was a pause, and then the voice said, "I'm sorry, what building are you in?"

Tom tried to sound impatient. "The new one. I'm in the basement, of all the God forsaken areas. Are you going to finish this or what?"

After another pause, the voice said, "When do you need it?"

"Now," Tom responded, "I need it now, and I have a list of equipment in case you've lost yours."

"Bring the list by," the voice said after a pause, and then added, "Who does this get billed to?"

"I told you," Tom said with irritation, "Dr. Blackwell. I'll bring the list over, but I'm moving in right now, and I could use some help."

"I'll send someone over."

For the next several days Tom busied himself with unpacking equipment and setting up his stolen lab. The space was perfect. Even though there were no views or windows, there was privacy, and Tom had come to realize that privacy was a greater commodity than any penthouse suite. Let the others fight over corner offices, he thought, the more windows and views, the more eyes upon you, and the less you will be able to focus on your work.

When Dr. Blackwell returned from his trip, he spent several days catching up. By the time he found Tom, there were already experiments under way in the new lab.

Dr. Blackwell surveyed the equipment with appreciation, and then asked Tom what he was working on.

"Phosphenes," Tom said, "The lights you see dancing in front of your eyes when someone hits you in the head."

"Ah," Richard said. Then after a pause, "Are you going to be able to find the visual detection threshold that the Navy wants?"

"Well…" Tom replied, "It will take a lot of work, and I could use some help."

Dr. Blackwell wrung his hands, "I'm behind, Tom. The Navy is getting anxious. They discovered in World War Two that one of the problems they had in launching torpedoes is that the seaman responsible for spotting a submarine could mistake it for a wave, a whale or any other number of things. They need hard evidence on what the human eye can perceive, and without solid research results, I could lose the funding."

Dr. Blackwell was approaching the point where he had to produce, and he lacked the finesse to construct the right experiments to do it.

Tom considered for a moment, and then responded, "I need help. Specifically, I need Russ DeValois and Tanner, if they're available."

Dr. Blackwell thought for a brief moment, then made a mental calculation of the funds available, and said, "Call them and see if you can bring them on board. I'll hire them too, but you'll have to produce something significant within three months. After that, we'll all be on our own. By the way, did you happen to check in with Dr. Girrard when you arrived?"

"Girrard? No," Tom answered.

"He *is* the director of the lab facilities on campus," Blackwell continued, "Are you sure this space was available?"

"Sure," said Tom, "It was empty and not even set up. They probably were just going to use it for storage."

Blackwell considered for a moment, then turned and left.

Before the door had closed, Tom was on the phone with Spike. When Spike answered Tom said, "You'll never guess who wants to hire you."

"Tom!" was the response, "Where are you? I thought you were at Hopkins!"

Tom smiled, it was good to hear Spikes voice. "I'm back," he said.

"Back where?"

"Back at Michigan."

"What the hell are you doing there?" Spike shot to Tom.

"Spending Dr. Blackwell's money," Tom said, "Want to help me? For that matter, do you know if Russ is finished with his Fullbright? We could all three go through a ton of Dr. Blackwell's funding."

Spike laughed, "Of course! That makes perfect sense! You're back at

Michigan and seeking revenge!"

"No, not really," Tom said in a serious tone, "Richard really needs the help, and I have a full lab set up. We can work on his project, and probably, if we are clever enough, we can do some other interesting things."

Spike thought for a moment, and then said, "Of course I want to come along. I'll see if I can get in touch with Russ. He should be finishing up. I can't believe it. We can raise hell again at Michigan."

When Russ arrived at Michigan he began his search for Tom and Spike. He knew to avoid the traditional established offices, neither Tom nor Spike would be found in such places. It took him only a little more than an hour to explore a doorway into an unmarked lab in a basement where he found Tom and Spike bent over equipment.

"Welcome!" Tom said as he spotted Russ, "You found us!"

"Wasn't hard," Russ said, "I just followed my nose to the stench of rat urine."

"No doubt." Tom smiled. "How was your 'Fullbright'?"

Russ paused, "It was fine. I spent the time in Germany."

"So we hear," Spike interjected, "But what exactly were you doing with all the money they gave you?"

Russ became even more uneasy and fidgeted before he answered. "I published a great work on geotropisms," he said and added, "in German."

"Of course," Tom said, as he came around the table closer to Russ. Tom and Spike knew that Russ was uneasy. They had learned to read him over the years, and were not about to let him off that easily.

"Geotropisms in what?" Tom asked.

"Beetles," Russ answered, and then attempted to change the subject by admiring some new equipment.

"What kind of beetles?" Spike asked.

"The kind that moves objects along mathematical planes..." Russ murmured.

"But," Tom continued, "Exactly what *kind* of beetle moves objects along mathematical planes?" Tom and Spike were grinning, and Russ was looking down.

"Dung beetles," Russ finished.

"Dung beetles?" Tom said, "You spent two years in Germany working with – let me get this straight – bugs that lay their eggs in shit?"

"Fine!" Russ shot back, "So it wasn't Nobel Prize material! No one there complained about it, so I don't know why you two are so critical!"

Spike and Tom were laughing. They knew that Russ had basically taken two years to have fun, and the fact that they could embarrass him over it was the icing on the cake.

"Never mind, Russ," Tom said in conciliatory tones, "We won't ask you to unclog the plumbing if it stops up. Even if you are, among the three of us, the dung expert."

"Yeah, well thanks," Russ responded, moving the conversation along, "Now, what are we doing here?"

"Welcome to the new visual physiology lab!" Tom exclaimed, "We were recently discovered by the department of ophthalmology, and they have several things they want us to do, but we also report to Dr. Blackwell in his visual detection project."

"Blackwell still hasn't found it?" Russ asked incredulously.

"My job," Spike said, "I'm to find the visual threshold for Blackwell."

"And then what?" Russ asked, "What are we supposed to be working on after that?"

Tom contemplated for a moment. "I have a probe," he said. "We made it at Hopkins, and I can reach any portion of the brain you want."

Russ was quiet, then asked, "What do you plan to go after?"

"The hypothalamus. I found an interesting thing at Hopkins. Did you happen to read about the experiment involving the amygdala?" Tom asked.

"The one about the anger center?" Russ asked, "Sure, it was in several journals."

"That was Bard and Hardcastle," Tom said.

"From here?" Russ said, "The guys from Michigan?"

"Johns Hopkins made Vernon Hardcastle the Dean of their school four years ago, so naturally he brought Phillip Bard and Jersey Rose on board," Tom continued.

"They were the ones to design the experiment, and shortly after they used my probe to get to the amygdala, we found the part of the brain that controls mating behavior, the hypothalamus."

"Whew!" Russ said, "Well it had to be somewhere. But I haven't read about it. Did you publish?"

"Not yet," Tom said, "I didn't have time. But I want to continue with that research here."

"What about administration? You know old Ralph Girrard will have a heart attack if he knows you are studying *anything* that has the word sex attached to it – even if it's the brain.'"

"He doesn't have to know," Tom said, "We're hard to find here. Besides, we answer to Blackwell, and all he cares about is Spike getting the military off his back."

"OK," Russ said, "Visual research first, then we play."

"Exactly," Tom replied.

For two months the three finished the lab, complete with surgical operatories. They were organized and clean, and as Dr. Blackwell occasioned in, he was impressed. He noticed that frequently there would be an outstanding amount of equipment that seemed to be dedicated to neurological research, and not visual research, but the papers were flowing nicely from Spike, and the Navy was pleased so far.

Dr. Blackwell had the good sense to leave the three alone – after all, they required almost no direction or prodding, and his precious funding was intact.

As the mapping of the brain continued, Tom and Russ began to realize that all of the structures were interrelated. As a probe neared a single brain cell, the loud speakers that hung on the walls of the operatory registered a steady popping sound. It was the background metabolism of the cell, and it fired at a steady rate. When the probe was advanced into the cell it made a loud bang, after which the cell sealed itself around Tom's microelectrode, and the steady popping sound resumed.

It startled Dr. Girrard once, who had caught wind of the excellent results and publications from the new visual physiology lab. He walked in one day just as Tom was in surgery and had nearly finished placing a probe. Girrard had taken an immediate dislike to Tom. *He* was supposed to be running this lab, along with several others, but Tom had never approached him or even remotely attempted to go through proper channels. Girrard could do nothing about it, as the various departments were excited about the work Tom was doing. Knowing this only served to anger him more.

One day he decided to make a call on the lab with the intention of keeping his presence known. It would serve well to remind Tom that he was under scrutiny. As he opened the door to the lab, the probe Tom had been placing penetrated the single cell, causing the speakers to protest with a loud bang.

"What the hell was that?" Girrard exclaimed.

Tom glanced up from the surgery, "Out!" he said, "No one is allowed in here!"

Girrard started, and then with a mixed emotion of shock and

embarrassment, retreated out the door.

"He doesn't like you," Russ said from the back of the lab. Tom grunted and continued with the surgery. Girrard would eventually find a way to make things difficult, he thought, but it would take him a while. Meanwhile, he was on to something.

"OK," he said, "I have the probe set where I want it. This time we measure the cells' metabolism while the female rat is stimulated sexually."

Russ coughed and Spike looked up from his microscope.

"And just how are we going to do that?" Russ asked, "She's out cold. No male rat will have anything to do with her."

Tom looked over to Spike who said, "Don't look at me, I have a girlfriend." Tom smiled, Spike was short and heavy and basically belligerent.

"I bet your girlfriend can't hold a candle to this rat," he said.

"Forget it," Spike said, then returned to his work.

"Look," Tom said, "It's simple. Any tactile stimulus in the general area should work. We are only trying to see what happens to the brain cells." With that, he used a small swab to gently massage the female rat. Immediately the frequency over the loudspeaker changed. Instead of the steady background idle, there emitted a higher frequency signal.

"Ah," Russ observed, "I think she wants you, Tom."

"Shut up," Tom rejoined, and then said, "Her brain is intrinsically linked to her reproductive system, as I suspect it is with all animals."

Russ was still in a joking mood, "So the only trick to getting a date for Spike is to set a few brain probes in a girl?"

"If you could be serious for a moment," Tom said, "I want to take this a little further. We need to inject her with estrogen. If my theory is correct, it will potentiate the brain signals."

"Can't," Russ said, "All hormones are insoluble in the blood stream. There's no way to get a solution into her."

"We did it at Hopkins," Tom said, "All we need to do is break up the solution into microscopic crystals using ultrasound."

"You really *were* working at Hopkins," Russ said in German.

Spike looked up, "That's beetle talk," he said. Then to Tom, "Russ has learned to speak to the dung beetles about where to roll their manure."

As Russ commented back to Spike in French expletives, Tom prepared the solution and injected it. The female rat brain now took on a new rhythm. There was a steady background noise overlaying the basic firing of the neuron. When she was physically stimulated again, the noise filled the room, and

Tom was jubilant. "I knew it!" he exclaimed.

"What?" Spike and Russ said in unison.

"What do you think?" Tom said, "The brain is the center for reproduction, not the ovaries, not the uterus, not any other of the apparatus associated with mating. The *brain!*"

Russ and Spike were silent. After a pause, Russ said, "So where does this get us?"

"Don't you see?" Tom flared, "In undergrad and even graduate school, our psychology professors claimed that the mechanisms of the brain had nothing to do with human or animal behavior. They adamantly stuck to the idea that all we needed to know about what makes us act in certain ways is observed through the actions, as if they were totally independent of the physiology of the person."

"Yeah, well," Spike said, "I think I said it best in personality theory to Blackie. 'This is all bullshit!'" Spike was still proud of the memory.

"Well, Spike, now we have proof," Tom said.

"OK," Russ said, "So what do we do with it? How does this affect anything?"

Tom turned to him and said, "Think for a moment," he paused, "Think about the treatments for debilitating mental diseases. How much progress is being made in the treatment of schizophrenia, for example? What about autism? What about affective disorders such as paranoia and suicide? Has modern medicine made significant progress in treating these diseases? How can it if the workings of the brain are not even considered relevant?"

Russ and Spike listened with interest. "You're starting to sound like a clinician," Spike said, "I thought you hated that idea."

Tom gathered himself from his passionate statements. "I hate the fact that most clinicians will not listen to us," he said, "But I do want to help people. I just don't care for the politics involved."

Russ and Spike nodded. "Hence," Spike said, "Our own little island here in the basement where nobody bothers us."

"Right," Tom said, then prepared to revive the rat.

Tom was ever so careful in his surgeries. A professor who said Tom would never be able to conduct animal brain surgeries without introducing infection had challenged him once. To this day, Tom had never allowed one of the animals to become contaminated. His operatory was kept sterile to a fanatical degree. This rat would be gently revived, and when she recovered, there would be no trauma. She would live a normal rat life, carrying only a small scar on her scalp from the delicate surgery. A testimony to a sacrifice she had unwillingly made, but one that would hopefully reduce the suffering of the species that held her in captivity.

Dr. Ian Behrman was a renowned obstetrician, as well as a researcher, yet his notoriety had taken him in a direction he never would have anticipated. Post war America was in a frenzy of domestic nurturing. It was almost as if the population was determined to replenish itself following the loss of thousands of young men in the Second World War. It was also a time of affluence and stability, and family values centered on a groomed lawn for children to engage in their own activities.

Unfortunately, not every family was able to have children, and that's where Dr. Behrman entered the picture. His medical clinic was the foremost leading center for infertility, and hundreds of patients anxiously awaited his solutions to their empty nests. He had a large degree of success. Some of the patients had simple problems that could easily be overcome. Those were the most rewarding cases, as the patients treated him like a miracle worker when, in fact, he had only made a minor correction. A few patients were untreatable due to serious disorders. Occasionally the male was infertile, and the family would be compassionately directed to caseworkers that counseled on adoption. Some patients, however, were an enigma. The sperm count was high enough in the father, ovulation occurred on time and the egg was fertile, and there were no blockages in the cervix to prevent the sperm from reaching its destination.

Dr. Behrman had learned to be tactful in his questioning, but still he needed answers. "When did you last have intercourse?" he would calmly ask a young woman.

"Yesterday," she would nervously respond, "and the day before and the day before that." She would blurt out.

"How long since your last cycle?" Dr. Behrman would continue.

"Nine days," she would respond.

"Well, it should work then." Dr. Behrman said in his most calming tone, "You just have to have patience."

"But Doctor Behrman!" the woman would exclaim, "This has been going on for months! Lydia next door is pregnant with her *second* child, and we were married at the same time! What is *wrong* with me..." she would trail off.

I don't know, Dr. Behrman thought to himself, but it's nothing physical, at least not that I can find.

Then he would offer some palliative treatment, mostly to keep the woman's hopes up, and possibly to cover the fact that he hadn't a clue what was wrong.

Dr. Behrman had friends on the faculty at Michigan's medical school. He wasn't particularly close to them, but on occasion he would join them at a club after work hours for a drink.

One evening, he walked in to see several of his colleagues sitting at a nearby table, and as he approached he caught a portion of the conversation.

"...sexual studies, I'm telling you. He's doing it on rats, but he is supposed to be working for the ophthalmology department," one of the professors was saying.

"I remember him from the graduate school," another speaker said.

"He was a royal pain in the ass..." at which point the first speaker looked up and noticed the smiling face of Dr. Berhman.

"Oh, hi, Ian," he said, "Have a seat."

Ian sat down, and then asked, "Who's doing sex studies without my knowing about it?" The professors at the table laughed nervously. They were uncomfortable discussing the topic in general, and they were particularly sensitive to the fact that Ian Behrman was tainted in his own way. The fact that he was an obstetrician kept him more or less respectable in their eyes, but still, he worked on the fringe.

"Oh," one professor started, "nobody Ian. Just a radical young scientist with absolutely no respect for anyone or anything."

"Who?" Ian pressed.

"Law," he responded, "His name is Tom Law. Works in the new visual research lab and is supposed to stick to vision research, but that idiot Blackwell lets him do anything he wants."

"What, exactly, is Tom Law doing?" Ian asked, trying to not sound overly interested.

"We're not exactly sure, Ian, but he has recently returned from a post doc at Hopkins. They made a special probe up there, and this guy Law thinks he has found a sexual center, but get this, he thinks it is in the *brain*!"

The other professors laughed.

Ian chuckled along with them, then said "Well, all I can tell you is that the brain is as good a place as any to look. Some of my patients are hiding it from me, and that's about the only place left to look." The table became uncomfortable with the direction the conversation was taking, and one of them rapidly changed the topic to matters of government spending and how it should be easy to garner grant money, if you had the right connections.

Ian spent some friendly time with his colleagues, then bade them goodnight and left. He was thinking about the rebellious scientist they mentioned. There were two types of rebellion in researchers; one that stemmed from not being able to handle structure, and one that arose out of frustration at the myopic stupidity of ones contemporaries. He was curious which of these two Tom Law would be.

Ian found Tom the next day at his lab. When he walked in, he immediately appreciated the sterile and organized surgeries. Even though this was just an animal lab, it was something that rivaled hospitals in attention to detail and cleanliness. Also, it was obvious, some money had been spent.

Tom looked up from his desk and asked, "Yes? Is there something I can help you with?"

"Maybe," Ian responded, "I'm looking for Dr. Law. Can you tell me where to find him?"

Tom looked straight into his eyes and said, "Who wants to find him, …and why?"

Ian smiled and offered his hand. "I'm Dr. Ian Behrman. I run a fertility clinic that you may have heard about." Tom accepted the hand and smiled back.

"I'm Tom."

Ian shook Tom's hand and said, "Yes, I gathered that. The faculty says you have an attitude." Ian was still smiling, and his demeanor suggested he held secrets from administration also. Tom instantly made the decision to trust him, although he wasn't completely sure why.

"I've heard of your clinic, Dr. Behrman. But you're treating human patients, so I'm wondering what brings you to this lab. As you can see, we are limited to rats in our explorations." Tom smiled.

Dr. Behrman asked if he could have a seat, and Tom indicated a chair. After they were settled, Dr. Behrman cleared his throat and began carefully.

"It's frustrating, Dr. Law, to look into the face of a patient who is pleading with you, and then have to tell her that there is nothing wrong with her physically, but for some reason she cannot get pregnant. And unfortunately, there are a lot of them in my practice. All physical exams turn up absolutely nothing. Month after month they come back to me, and every time they expect me to tell them that they're pregnant or that I have the cure for their infertility.

Hopeful young women with watery eyes and down turned mouths, their husbands waiting for news and, of course, their parents wringing their hands in anticipation of grandchildren. Some of these young women are desperate. All of them are despondent, and it grieves me for them. Also, I admit, I'm losing confidence in myself. I *should* be able to find *something*."

Tom looked at the older man. He had never spent much time with clinicians, but he had taught medical students many times in the past. The best doctors were the ones that suffered for their patients; it was a more important attribute than intelligence. He decided that Dr. Behrman was both compassionate and bright. Otherwise, he would simply write off a portion of his patients as unresponsive to treatment and spend less time thinking about them than he spent thinking about a new set of golf clubs.

"I'm still not sure what brings you here," Tom said, "This is the visual physiology lab." "So I gathered," Ian said, "But there are rumors…" he trailed off.

"Who's talking?" Tom asked flatly.

"I'll be honest with you, Tom," Ian said, "I overheard a conversation some of the medical school faculty were having about you last night. They were discussing your 'extra-curricular' activities on the brain."

"Which faculty members?" Tom asked, and Ian listed the names. Tom sighed. Word certainly spread fast, especially if there was a potential for scandal. Well, he thought, at least Girrard had not caught wind of it yet. Or, if he had, he was not taking it too seriously.

"OK," Tom said to Ian, "So I have a theory about the brain, and the control it exerts on the organism."

"Go on," Ian said, paying special attention now. Tom described his experiments in detail, including some of the foundations that had been laid back at Hopkins. He concluded with a jubilant statement on the hypothalamus and the potentiation of the neurons with either hormones or with tactile stimulation, or most of all, with both combined.

Ian looked at Tom with a blank expression, then said, "I'm following you, sort of, so let me see if I am understanding what you're saying."

Tom looked at Ian and waited patiently.

"You're saying, that besides the brain controlling the *physical* aspects of our bodies, such as respiratory rate and other autonomic functions, it's in essence, controlling the behavioral aspects of our bodies. Aspects that heretofore were relegated to the field of psychology. Is that it?"

"Yes!" Tom exclaimed, "You get it!"

"Well," Ian said, "I understand what you're saying, Tom, but I can't honestly say I'm convinced it's true." Tom looked chagrined.

Then Ian hastily added, "OK. I admit what you found is a breakthrough. But you're extrapolating a lot. Take my personal problem, for instance. How does your theory affect my patients?"

"I don't know," Tom said with some irritation, "You're the physician, not me. But I'll offer this much to you. I'm willing to bet that fully ten percent of your female patients who are 'infertile' do not enjoy sex with their partners."

Ian's eyebrows shot up in surprise. "What could that possibly have to do with it?" he asked.

"The brain," Tom said, "If I'm right, then the brain has a lot to do with reproduction. Or, to paraphrase it, there is a lot more to reproduction than just the physical and mechanical actions."

"Go on," Ian prompted.

"Reproductive behavior is complex in higher organisms," Tom continued, "We're a far cry from cell division as a means to propagate ourselves. Even rats seem to have a social structure of sorts, but humans, well, our selection process is *very* complicated. The way a woman selects a man as a mate is the endless subject of debate, or the way a man selects a woman for that matter. So, we have to ask ourselves, what changes in higher organisms? It is not the basic machinery. Our sperm and eggs are not all that different from those of sea urchins. What *has* changed is brain size and complexity. So my suggestion, Dr. Berhman, is that your female patients are not happy with their selections, and as a result, something is preventing them from becoming pregnant."

Ian contemplated Tom's statement for a while, and then said, "I'll look into it. Maybe some form of cervical eclampsia is taking place and keeping the sperm out. At the very least, Tom, this has been fascinating. I wish you the best in your research." Ian smiled, shook hands, and left the lab. Tom thought about it for a moment. He wondered if he was right or just fighting status quo for the sake of it. No, he thought, I am right. Nothing else makes sense.

Two weeks later, Ian found Tom again at the lab. He swung the door open, found Tom behind a partition sitting at a desk and took a seat opposite him.

Ian was beaming. "Would you believe fifty percent?" he said. Then, in response to the blank look on Tom's face, "Fifty percent of the infertile female patients fit your profile. You are right. They are somehow mentally blocking fertilization."

Tom smiled back. "Really! How did you find out?"

"Well," Ian continued, "It's a delicate matter, and you certainly don't want to interview the patient with her husband in the same room. But these women, if you ask the right questions, all admit to finding the entire sexual act repulsive. Not a single one of them will ever climax and that can be a large part of the mystery. Without the cervical response to orgasm, the architecture is not in place or at least it is not optimized. At any rate, we are back to your brain and the intricacies involved with intercourse."

Tom was excited. This was the first validation he had experienced from anyone outside of himself. Here was a notable physician who not only accepted Tom, but he had the means to carry the research into useful application.

"What do you plan to do?" Tom asked.

"Set up another clinic," Ian responded, "But I need one away from my practice, and I could use some expert help." Ian was looking at Tom and gauging his response.

"Here," Tom said, "We have room and equipment. But," he added, "We don't have much funding or personnel. You'll have to provide the bodies."

"Done," Ian said, and then left Tom with the promise he would return soon.

For the next two weeks, the lab was in constant turmoil. Spike had recently completed the research Dr. Blackwell required for the Navy contract, and lacking the enthusiasm for Tom's reproductive studies, took his leave of his friends. Russ remained, however, and together with Tom he modified a portion of the visual detection lab that had been Spike's home. Dr. Berhman required unusual equipment. It made Russ queasy to install the beds that were to be used by female patients. Both he and Tom, in fact, spent a lot of time looking over their shoulders as the lab was modified, for fear of a faculty member catching wind of the project. Dr. Behrman was confident, however.

"You are only fifty yards from the medical clinic," he said, "And there's nothing more noble than helping human patients."

"That's fine," Tom said, "But my doctorate is a PhD, not MD. If it's all the same to you, we'll stay out of the quarters. I can help with setting up the experiments, but for the sake of my sanity and reputation, we will never, ever, enter into the patients' area."

"A wise decision, Tom," Ian said, then clapped a friendly hand on Toms shoulder. "You and Russ remain outside. You can help us quantify our results, and I'll see to it your name is on every publication."

Tom considered that and felt mixed emotions. On the one hand, this was potentially a medical breakthrough. On the other, appearances were everything. He had been flying under the radar so far in his basement, but prudery was irrational, and he had plenty of enemies already.

"Thanks, Ian," he said, "When it gets to that point, let me consider it. I'm not sure if the notoriety will necessarily help my career, but I appreciate the offer."

"As you wish," Ian responded.

For the next six weeks Tom slept very little, if at all. He spent much of his time nervously fiddling with an experiment on the periorbital potentials of the eye that he and Russ recorded, but his mind was ever drawn to the adjacent lab. In there, he knew, were young women who wanted to become pregnant. All other means having been exhausted, they reverted to the final recourse of reconditioning their minds. This reconditioning was, in all reality, a form of sexual stimulation.

The results so far were encouraging. Using apparatus that Tom had dutifully designed, the women were instructed in relaxation techniques coupled with self stimulation. Tom wanted to remain as aloof as possible, yet it was largely his responsibility to set up the laboratory equipment. He cringed at the thought that he, himself, had designed the vaginal insert that could be inflated to various dimensions using a valve. The idea was simple, create the ideal penis, and let the female patient be the judge as to just what that entailed. He didn't want to think about it, but there was a need to make a valve that would inflate the device and that could be easily controlled by the patient, yet all he could come up with was the valve on the French horn. Tom had played the instrument before, but he could not remember what had happened to it. So for lack of better direction, he found a pawnshop and purchased a French horn for $50 and expensed it on his lab budget.

When accounting called him into the office and asked him to explain why he needed a French horn in his lab, he was evasive.

"I just needed it," he said.

"For what?" the young woman with large brown eyes asked, "Music?"

"No. Not for music," Tom said, "Research."

"You are researching using music?" she said in a dulcet voice.

"Look," Tom said, "I just needed it. Believe me when I tell you, you don't want to know the details."

And with that Tom turned around and walked out, leaving the bemused accountant to decide just how to expense it.

As the young female patients in the lab were conditioned to become more relaxed and receptive to coitus, they became more receptive to the act of intercourse. Progress was being made, and while it was logical and the natural extrapolation of Tom's theories, it left him in a constant state of agitation. Dr. Behrman was used to human patients, but Tom had only worked on animals. It shouldn't make a difference, and if anything, it was more ethical to provide therapy to willing humans than to work on captive lab animals, but some of the existing cultural prudery seeped into Toms mind, and his brief dreams at night were haunting.

Russ was no better off. He had taken to avoiding the lab, and instead spent much of his time keeping Blackwell busy and away. The ophthalmology department required handling as well, since they lay claim to nearly fifty percent of the funding for this lab. Tom was visibly nervous, but Dr. Behrman, who kept a small office adjacent to the research lab, was jubilant.

"This is major, Tom," he would say, "Who knows how far and wide this sort of problem runs? These are only the patients desperate enough to present themselves to my clinic. I know that when word gets out that there is hope, hundreds more will surface."

Tom tried to look happy, but all he could manage was a weak smile.

"Cheer up, Tom!" Ian said, "Soon we'll have a mountain of evidence, and you're responsible for helping potentially hundreds of families realize their dreams."

"That's fine," Tom said, "But I...." Tom's sentence was interrupted by the main door to the lab bursting open.

Three men stood in the doorway; the first was the director, Ralph Girrard, followed by two other faculty members. Girrard strode forward.

"What the HELL is going on here!"

Dr. Behrman stood up and faced the man. "Research," he said, "and if I may be so bold, it's on the forefront of medical science."

"Get out of my way!" Girrard continued, "Law! You're responsible for this, aren't you?"

Ian again attempted to address Girrard, "Dr. Law has graciously loaned us a portion of the facility, but this is my program."

Girrard regarded Ian. "And who the hell are you?"

"I'm Dr. Behrman," Ian said, "I'm an obstetrician. I run a medical clinic nearby."

"Oh yes, I have heard of you," Girrard raged, "You run the sex clinic."

"Fertility clinic," Ian corrected, "And we run a respectable..."

"To hell with you and your clinic!" Girrard interrupted. Ian was becoming angry, but fought to control it.

"Now listen," he said, "You should be grateful for what we're doing. It's entirely at my expense, yet your university will only benefit as a result."

Ralph Girrard stood and looked at him. "Not," he said, "In.... MY Medical School!"

The two men stood facing one another, then after a moment, Ian said, "Fine. I'll be out of here within two days."

Tom and Ian watched as Girrard and his company left, slamming the door behind them. Ian regarded Tom.

"Sorry," he said, "I had no idea...he should be grateful..." he trailed off.

"What will you do?" Tom asked.

"Move. We'll move and continue. You're welcome to join us, Tom."

Tom hesitated as he considered it. He knew this incident was only going to make matters worse for him here, but he didn't feel at home in a medical clinic.

"Thanks," he said, "But you really don't need me. You can finish all of this on your own. Besides, I am a theorist, not a clinician. It would always be uncomfortable for me."

Ian smiled a half smile, then turned away and began informing his staff of the situation. Within one day the facility was vacated, and Tom and Russ were left alone. Tom was relieved, but couldn't help but feel a sense of loss. He knew that Dr. Behrman would make history, if only a research facility would give him the chance.

Later that year, Tom learned that Dr. Behrman had been contacted by Ohio State University. They offered him a full professorship, plus an entire department complete with research facilities. Tom didn't correspond with Ian, but he heard that the clinic became famous, as did Dr. Behrman himself. Tom was happy for Ian, but mostly he hoped that the information he had learned of made its way back to Girrard.

Tom found the incident intolerable and wanted to punish the university in some way for their short sightedness, yet as myopic as the university was, he could not fault them entirely for clinging to their principles.

Tom was unprepared for the information he received several days later. It came about in an unusual manner. A publication mentioned Tom as the primary researcher in an experiment involving human subjects, patients that had no connection to Tom, but who had been reputedly diagnosed as nymphomaniacs. The publication, authored by a group of neurosurgeons, stated that due to the brain research of a Dr. Law, the reproductive center of the brain had been found and females suffering from nymphomania had been altered surgically and rendered "cured." "In fact," the journal went on, "The patients had undergone the surgery and their sexual drives had not only been cured, they had been eliminated altogether."

Tom read the remarks in disbelief and shook with rage. After finding a phone, he contacted the receptionist for the head surgeon of the study and was placed on hold. When the doctor came to the phone Tom laid in.

"This is Dr. Law," Tom said.

"Why hello, Dr. Law," the voice answered, "Glad to actually speak with you."

"First of all," Tom began, "You will immediately desist with this butchery. And second, if you do not, I will discredit you and all of your staff for the mutilation of helpless women."

There was a pause, then the voice said, "I don't understand. You yourself discovered the points of the brain that enabled us to cure these women. I would think you would be happy that we mentioned you in our publication."

Tom breathed in, then said, "I do not ever, ever advocate mutilating a human mind in this manner. Is that clear? The purpose of my research is to find the *functional* centers of the brain. This is not to suggest that you can wantonly create lesions in those centers to your own twisted perceptions of propriety. Who are you to offer the diagnosis of nymphomania? Worse yet, now that you have eliminated the possibility of these hapless women ever having children, how do you reconcile the lost future generations that they might have had?!" Furious still, Tom continued. "You have dabbled in a genetic breeding program commensurate with the Nazi's of World War Two. If you continue, I swear, I *will* discredit you, and at the very least, I will quit my research and end all projects that could enable you to do more harm."

After a long pause, the doctor said, "OK. OK, Dr. Law, point made."

Tom hung up the phone and sat down heavily. Things were not going in the direction that he had planned. All of this was far beyond his worst imaginings.

For the next several months, Tom continued with optical research. For the time being, he decided to give up on his studies of reproductive behavior. The incident with Dr. Behrman was a painful reminder that he could not ignore the political structure of the university. He regrouped, in a diligent yet disinterested way with Russ, and they published papers on night vision and electro stimulation of the eye, often using themselves as the subjects of the studies. It was enough to keep Dr. Blackwell happy, as well as the department of ophthalmology, but it was becoming repetitive and boring.

Tom made a point of spending some time with friends intending to relax, but instead found himself complaining about the political machinery of the university, and the basic incompetence of politicians in general. Tom was in the middle of one of these lengthy dissertations one day over lunch with his attorney friend Peter Darrow, when Peter looked up and said, "If you're really as sick of the system as much as you say you are, why not do something about it, instead of endlessly gripping?"

Tom started for a moment, and then said, "Right. I'll win the faculty's love and take over the medical school."

Peter chuckled, "No. I'm serious. I think you should run for the Senate."

Tom nearly spit out the sandwich he had been chewing on, "Senate?" he said, "What did you put in your ice tea, Peter?"

"OK," Peter said, "It's like this. Our incumbent senator has been in office for years and wins by a landslide every time. The truth is, no one wants to run against him. This is a conservative state, and he's extremely popular. You'd be nothing more than a sacrificial lamb. Just a name to put on the ballot to make the election legal."

Amused by the thought, Tom said, "You've already thought this through, haven't you?"

Peter smiled, "Well, you can take the challenge or you can continue to sit around whining about everything." Tom chewed the rest of his sandwich in contemplation. "Don't worry. Tom," Peter said, "You're going to lose by fifteen points at the minimum. All you have to do is agree to it, and I'll make the arrangements."

For a moment, Tom thought about the medical school and the implications there. Normally, he would never agree to anything that removed him from his precious lab and research, but lately he had become more than a little disillusioned.

"OK," he said, "But let me get permission from the school first. I'm being watched very closely these days, and I'm treading on thin ice."

"Let me know," Peter said amiably.

One week later, Tom called Peter and said it was a go.

Tom couldn't believe it himself when the first person he approached, Ralph Girrard, gave his permission. It made Tom suspicious, so he continued on up the chain of command at the university. The next person he approached was the director of the Mental Health Institute, the person that Girrard answered to directly. Permission was again granted. Tom, still in disbelief approached the director of the ophthalmology department, and finally the Dean of the medical school.

From the Dean, he actually extracted the permission in writing, so he could show it to the others in case their memories needed reminding.

Peter said that Tom's name was to be placed on the ballot and thanked Tom for doing his patriotic duty.

"That's it?" Tom asked Peter.

"That's it, Tom," Peter said, "You can go back to your lab and your rats now."

Tom hung up the phone and thought about the election. It would be a shame really, to not give the incumbent a good race. But to organize a campaign of this magnitude would require considerable funds. Something that researchers were known to lack. His salary barely covered his meager existence. Probably, he surmised, campaign contributions were easy to come by if you supported big business. Large corporations needed tax laws that were friendly to them, and Michigan had a host of huge companies. No, he thought, this would never be a fair fight. Tom was close to letting it go, to returning to his lab and the career for which he had trained all these years.

Yet when Peter Darrow placed the announcement in the papers the following day, all hell broke loose on campus. Tom was called into the offices of each person who had given him permission, and starting with Ralph Girrard, every one of them demanded that Tom drop out of the race and retract his announcement in the paper.

"Why?" Tom asked Girrard, "You gave me permission."

"I don't give a damn about the permission," Girrard said, "You will retract immediately." Tom stood across the desk from Girrard and stared in disbelief and anger. He removed the written permission document and placed it on the desk for Girrard to see, but Girrard simply grabbed it, crumpled it and threw it in a wastebasket.

Tom shook with anger as he regarded the action. "I won't quit," he said with finality.

"Then," Girrard said, "As of right now, you are on a leave of absence. You don't work for us." Then, he added, to cover his legal obligation to the university, "This is an act of generosity on our part. You can dedicate yourself to the campaign. But as of now, the lab is no longer yours."

Tom stormed from the office and went straight to the Dean. Sitting opposite the Dean at his desk, Tom received a similar edict with the added statement that if he continued with the campaign, the Dean would see to it that Tom would never teach in a medical school again.

"Let me remind you that I have connections,"the Dean said, "Retract now, or there won't be one, single medical school in these United States that will hire you."

Tom left completely stunned. He struggled to find the logic of this sudden venomous turn, but he couldn't come up with anything. Perhaps, he thought, they hadn't known he would run as a democrat. But more likely, they had met together and discussed Tom's history with the administration. The possibility of him gaining political power in the Senate must have reminded them of the fact that Tom stuck to his ideals and would never be amenable to negotiation if it compromised something he believed in.

University funding was a state issue. Tom could conceivably end up in control of that. Yet, Tom thought, how could they seriously believe he had a chance of winning? The incumbent had been in office for forty years. The odds of unseating him were astronomically against Tom.

As he walked back to his office, he realized that his career at Michigan was over. Even if he retracted, the university was clearly against him. It had somehow become a personal issue, one that was out in the open now. Tom gathered his resolve. This would be a bloody battle.

One of the mistakes the university had made was letting Tom hire his own staff. Some were part-time but his secretary, a large black woman, was permanent. It was a time in which blacks were rarely hired in such a prestigious institution. Or, if hired at all, it was in a janitorial position, yet Tom didn't share their segregationist viewpoint. A person either had talent or they didn't. It mattered little to Tom what color they were, or if they were male or female. All that mattered was their willingness to help and to learn.

Bess had proven herself. She was brilliant, and Tom had become ever more dependant upon her. He found Bess at her desk, slowly packing her few personal effects into a cardboard box. Apparently, word had already reached her. She looked up at Tom with large, teary eyes and attempted a smile.

"They didn't offer to transfer you to another department?" Tom asked.

"Not a chance, Dr. Law," she said, "But even if they did, I wouldn't take it. No one outside of your lab treats me with respect. To them, I'm just an ignorant, black woman."

She finished with a tone of bitterness. "Ignorant hell," Tom said, "You know more about what's going on here than anyone else, including me!"

Bess smiled at Tom with tears in her beautiful eyes. He had been her champion and protector and she was uncertain what she would do now without him. Tom sat down heavily and regarded her. "I have an idea," he said, "I want you to be my campaign manager."

Bess shot a look at Tom. "Are you *serious*?" she said, "A black woman?"

"Totally serious," Tom said, "But there is a catch. I'm not sure I can pay you. In fact, we may both starve before the election ever gets here."

Bess's eyes lit up and she said, "Doesn't matter to me. It's not about the money. I'll find work at night if I have to."

Tom smiled and gave her a quick hug. "Welcome aboard," he said, "Again."

"Where do we start?" Bess said, she was quick to re-assess her situation.

"Gather anyone you can," Tom said, "But make sure they know this is 'pro bono' because our campaign contributions are likely to be nonexistent."

The next day, while Bess was making calls to an odd assortment of people, including the deacon of her all black church, Tom received and opened an envelope. It was addressed to the democratic senate party, but had arrived at Tom's home.

Inside was a check for one hundred dollars and a quick note that said simply, "Good luck." It was signed Anatol Rappaport. Tom nearly dropped the check. Anatol was a great mathematician who the university had proudly recruited a short while back. Well, Tom thought, I guess we have funding after all.

Bess kept herself busy recruiting help for the campaign. The first person she called was one of Tom's occasional contract employees, Vance. Tom had needed to find someone who could make instruments or prototypes out of a variety of materials, and Vance had come to the rescue. Vance could construct virtually anything, from blown glass containers to electrical circuits. As eccentric as they came, Vance amused everyone with his self proclaimed healthy lifestyle, living on soy products and rice.

He had a Masters Degree in math, yet disdained the establishment, and as such, was welcomed into Tom's lab. Vance and Bess determined that Tom needed a publicity manager, and after some investigation, found an English Professor who was not only friendly to Tom, but who offered to recruit heavily from the student body. While Bess continued to organize speaking engagements, Vance created car-top billboards and assembled them with the volunteer help of several students.

Tom stood in amazement of the entire process. He was surprised at the energy and dedication in his group. They required little or no direction from him, and in fact, it seemed they were far ahead of him in their vision for the election. Dr. Peterson, the new publicity manager, made it his job to create press releases. He was so prolific that one day, one of the local papers called him and asked how, exactly, Tom could manage to be in three separate speaking engagements on the very same afternoon.

Without hesitation Dr. Peterson said, "Oh well, my boy's pretty fast. He gets around like you wouldn't believe." There was a stunned silence on the other end of the phone. For once the reporter was without comment, causing Dr. Peterson to smile and wink at Tom who had just entered the room.

Not long after, it became a reality, as Tom did in fact, have several speaking engagements. The venue was odd in the fact that it ranged from gay rights meetings to the all-black churches that Bess facilitated. Everywhere, however, there was support.

Students on the campus as well as a good number of the employees carried the mobile billboards on the tops of their cars. Virtually everyone in the community that was not a solid republican aided in the burgeoning grass roots movement, and Tom allowed himself to actually grow hopeful. He had never believed that there would be a serious chance at winning, but the polls were steadily climbing in his favor.

The newspapers still gave only a minimal attendance to Tom's efforts until an incident happened that could not be ignored. A man who was nicknamed "Tiny" showed up at the campaign headquarters one day and said he wanted to help. Vance and Bess looked long and hard at the person standing in the doorway. He was about six feet, eight inches tall, a startling fact in and of itself.

"What do you want to do to help?" Bess asked.

"Anything," this giant of a man responded, "I don't really care, I just want Dr. Law to get the recognition he deserves."

Vance raised his eyebrows and with a kidding smile said, "Well, would you be willing to walk naked through the middle of Ann Arbor?"

Tiny just smiled.

The very next day the newspapers had photos on their covers featuring a very tall man walking down the street with a very short Dr. Law. The giant was wearing nothing but a barrel suspended by a strap over his shoulder and with a hanging banner that read, "The opponent put us in this barrel. Won't you help get us out?"

The Republican Party was indignant, and called Bess. "Dirty trick" was the term they used, along with several pointed threats.

Bess calmly waited for the speaker to finish, then asked, "Would your candidate like to have a debate with ours?"

"Any day," the angry voice said, "Any day, any time, you just name the place."

"I'll arrange it," Bess said, then hung up the phone.

Tom was not overly pleased at this engagement. Everyone knew that to challenge an incumbent in a debate was suicide. There were a myriad of issues that he would know nothing about and because of that, Tom could end up looking like a fool. Yet in the end, he acquiesced. He decided that to win a debate, he would have to expose the incumbent in some manner. A manner that hit close to home for the populace. One such issue was the educational budget. Tom knew that a lot of funding had been diverted from school cafeteria programs, and instead had been spent on other programs that lined the pockets of lobbyists.

When the debate occurred, the incumbent was trapped, and Tom gained momentum in the polls yet again. The day before election, Bess had borrowed a large convertible, and she and Tom drove around the city waving and smiling at the cheering crowds. A large black woman, and a small, white college professor were too much for the papers, and the polls moved from a five percent difference in favor of the incumbent, to a one percent difference.

Tom, after the tour, returned home and went straight to bed.

On Election Day, as the results were pouring in, the Democratic Committee sat in a circle watching anxiously. There was plenty of talk, but Tom quietly watched in fascination. When the polls closed and the final results were tallied, Tom found he had lost by one half of one percent. His staff and friends were disappointed, but not overly so. They felt that the effort had made history in a way and that they, themselves, were to a large extent responsible.

Tom thanked everyone, said that he would thank him or her more properly later and left.

When he arrived home his wife was standing at the door waiting for him. She had a worried look on her face and he could see she had been crying, but she tried to hide it. The twins, Michael and Daniel, were playing on the living room floor unaware of what was about to occur in their young lives.

"Tom, two men from the sheriff's department came by a little while ago. They left this message for you." She caught her breath and handed him an envelope. It was indeed, from the sheriffs department and it said; "We have been instructed to escort you to the border of Michigan State if you are not already gone by tomorrow morning."

Tom looked up from reading the letter at his teary eyed wife and said, "Pack up. We're leaving tonight."

"Where will we go?" she said through the tears that were flowing down her cheeks.

"California. I received a job offer out there a few months ago. I think I can still take it."

"Is it a medical school?" she asked hopefully, more for his sake than hers.

Tom snorted, "No. That's not likely to happen again. I guess I've offended just about everyone, particularly the medical school here. We're leaving, and not coming back."

He took his wife into his arms and together they walked back into the house toward their sons.

Tom, his wife, and both boys left in the middle of the night in an old flat bed truck he had borrowed from a friend and headed for California.

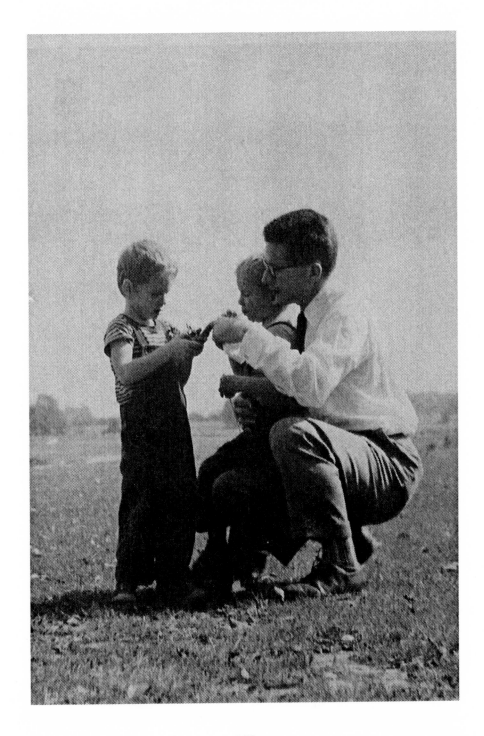

STATE LEGISLATURE

State Senate

O. THOMAS LAW

Tom Law would give Washtenaw County a forceful and progressive voice in the State Senate. A veteran and family man, Tom is a research worker at University Hospital. He believes in tax reform to provide funds for essential state services.

LEGISLATURE

1st. District

Annette C. Hodesh

Wife of a Ford Times Editor and mother of two boys. More interested in legislative accomplishment than personal promotion.

2nd. District

Maurice J. Hoffman

Sylvan Township Supervisor. Elected and re-elected because of service to his area.

U. S. CONGRESS

U. S. Congress

ROBERT G. HALL

Supt. of Schools, Cement City, Rural Agr. Schools, Lenawee County. Veteran and civic leader. Robert Hall will be a forceful and responsive spokesman for the Second District in Congress.

Vote November 4th

VOTE ☒ DEMOCRATIC !

ELECT THE SLATE
IN FIFTY-EIGHT

G. MENNEN WILLIAMS
(GOVERNOR)

JOHN B. SWAINSON
(LIEUTENANT GOVERNOR)

JAMES M. HARE
(SECRETARY OF STATE)

PAUL L. ADAMS
(ATTORNEY GENERAL)

SANFORD A. BROWN
(STATE TREASURER)

FRANK S. SZYMANSKI
(AUDITOR GENERAL)

PHILIP A. HART
(UNITED STATES SENATE)

ROBERT G. HALL
U. S. HOUSE OF REPRESENTATIVES)

O. THOMAS LAW
(STATE SENATE)

ANNETTE C. HODESH
(LEGISLATURE-FIRST DISTRICT)

MAURICE J. HOFFMAN
(LEGISLATURE-SECOND DISTRICT)

ROBERT GILLESPIE
(PROSECUTING ATTORNEY)

LAWRENCE OLTERSDORF
(SHERIFF)

ETHEL CLAIRE BROWN
(CLERK)

GARVIN J. BRASSEUR
(TREASURER)

ALICE CABLE HAYES
(REGISTER OF DEEDS)

EDWARD J. JONAS
(DRAIN COMMISSIONER)

WILLIAM LANTERMAN
(SURVEYOR)

REAL PROGRESS
IN MICHIGAN WITH
DEMOCRATIC
STATE OFFICERS

Let's Stop Drifting in
Washtenaw County!

ELECT DEMOCRATS ON
NOVEMBER 4th

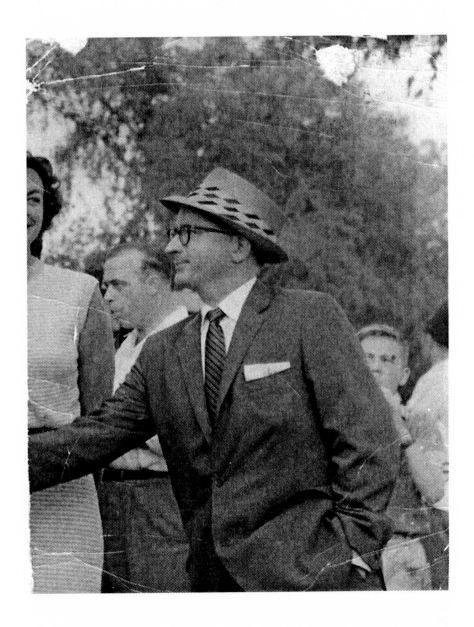

Chapter Eight

Put your hand out and you can feel
the warmth of working iron and steel

Tom arrived in California three days later and after stopping at a gas station, found the approximate location of the city of Downey. Autonetics Corporation had contacted Tom a few months before and flown a person out to interview him. Tom agreed to the interview, but didn't have the foggiest notion what this company wanted. From what he understood Autonetics manufactured missiles and were involved with military contracting.

He accepted the offer to interview in light of the hostile environment in which he found himself at the university, but he didn't really expect he would be taking a job with an engineering firm. He had asked the interviewer directly, "What in the world do you want with a Neurophysiologist in *your* industry?"

"Never mind," was the response, "We have our reasons." Tom was doubtful, but now he had nowhere else to turn. If the offer still stood, he would make a decent salary. Far better, in fact, than what he made as a professor or in research.

Tom found Autonetics following several frustrating side journeys, and after telling his wife he would be right back; he made his way to the personnel department where he was ushered into a waiting area and asked to take a seat. It wasn't long before the personnel director himself came out to greet Tom and invited him into his office.

"Thanks for coming," he said, "I can't tell you how glad we are to have you here."

Tom smiled and shook his hand. "Can you tell me what this is all about?" he asked, "What, exactly, is it that I could possibly do for you?"

"Before we begin," the director said, "I have to tell you something. You have the job. I told everyone that if you showed up within six months, we would hire you on the spot. You have an employee number, your own set of keys, everything, and nothing can change that. But I also want to tell you that a short while ago, your direct supervisor, a Dr. Girrard, called us and…well, said a few things."

Tom swallowed hard, then said, "I can only imagine."

The director smiled and continued. "Among other things, he said that you are a thief, a dishonest drunkard and a lot more that I don't care to mention. In short, he tried to bury you. You have a formidable enemy there."

Tom just shook his head and smiled, then said, "So, why am I hired?"

"Because, Tom," the director responded, "We checked you out. We have our sources, and you're none of those things."

Tom smiled and said, "I still don't know what I'm doing here, why do you want me? I'm a Neurophysiologist, not an engineer. Are you conducting some sort of animal tests?"

"Let me explain, Tom," the director said, "We have some problems here that we think you can help us solve. And no, we're not testing animals. We're building computer systems that aid in the guidance of our missiles, and frankly, the computer systems are becoming so complex that no one understands them.

It seems to us that they are becoming more and more like the human brain. We know that there are few people in the world that understand the brain as you do, and we know your expertise in electronics. We read your publications on the electro-surgical unit you perfected at Hopkins, and we're aware of the patent that you hold. We believe that your combination of skills is unique and… happens to be exactly what we need."

Tom was disillusioned; there was nothing that a computer had in common with a brain, much less a human brain. These people were either desperate or extremely naïve. However, he needed the job. He had arrived here in a broken down old truck that he had borrowed and little else. Even the few belongings he owned back at Michigan were still, for the most part, in their abandoned apartment.

He struggled with his conscience over the offer. He knew he could get several month's pay out of them before they let him go, when they realized that he knew nothing about missiles or their computers, but he would never be able to accept a position or assignment where he felt useless. It simply was not in his nature. The director was waiting for an answer.

"I'm not sure I can do what you ask," Tom said, "I don't know anything about your problems, nothing of your objectives, and I don't want to deceive you. I have to tell you that while I want to work here, there may be nothing of value that I have to offer."

"Relax, Tom," the director said, "We'll train you. At night you'll attend artillery school. During the day you'll help us with our project. This is the first artillery computer system ever designed; it's called the Field Artillery Digital Automatic Computer system or FADAC for short." He smiled and continued, "We've invested all our resources into this project, and I have to tell you, it's failing. Fifty percent of our missiles don't go where we want them to go and unless the problem is fixed soon, we won't get the military project." Tom started to speak, but the director cut him off. "Also," he said, "I need to tell you your position. You're the senior research engineer."

Tom returned to his wife who was sitting in the truck with the twins and told her the news. "On the plus side," he told her, "I have a job, and Autonetics has offered to move our belongings out to California, all the way down to the bricks that hold up our shelves and set us up in a place here. On the down side, I still haven't a clue what I'm to do for them."

Tom's wife breathed a heavy sigh of relief. After all that they had been through, the fact that Tom was momentarily directionless in his new job seemed of little importance. It was a new beginning, a new hope at a time where there had been none. Tom started the truck and headed for a motel where they could spend a few days and regroup.

Artillery school proved to be fascinating for Tom. It was basically physics, and he had little problem with that. What troubled him was the computer system he was supposed to be fixing during the days. The program was foreign to him, and while he studied to learn it, he kept coming up with the same conclusion as the other engineers, that obviously something was wrong. Missiles were launched from test sites, and nearly fifty percent of them ended up in the ocean. A few of them made such erratic turns that they threatened the observers who dove under cover and came out only after several anxious seconds that seemed to draw into hours.

At first, Tom believed that it was his ignorance in computers that was cursing the project, but after he gained some knowledge in programming, he realized that he understood what was supposed to be happening; yet there was something preventing it. At night, after artillery school, he laid in bed thinking. Countless times in the past he had experienced the same scenario. A surgery could take twelve to twenty hours to prepare, and yet when the critical moment came, the results were erratic or skewed. Often, he had found, it was a matter of checking and rechecking the equipment. With so many electrical components involved in probing the brain, there were bound to be errors. Sometimes the errors were as simple as a loose wire or a failed circuit breaker. Tom had learned to check each and every component in the experiments and often the problem was found and easily fixed. Over the past few years, however, he had become dependant on his staff to find and fix these problems.

Now it became his responsibility to find the solutions. If he understood the program right, it should be working. Perhaps it was wishful thinking, but maybe the problem was a simple one.

When Tom approached the computer system with his new perspective, he found several interesting things. The first and most rewarding was that some of the cables were faulty and could only carry the signal intermittently. Tom ordered all new cables and had every one replaced to his satisfaction. Yet, he found, the problem persisted. Not to the same degree, but there was still significant error. Something else must be the matter, he surmised, so he set about with his systematic detective work.

Ultimately he found the problem. The guidance systems were connected to the computers with a twelve-pin coupler. The twelve pins were set in an equidistant radial pattern, yet each pin carried different information. If the couple was placed in the wrong orientation, the information would be misread, and the missile launch would be disastrous. Tom couldn't believe it when he discovered this.

How stupid, he thought, that they would design a couple that *could* be placed wrong. This never would have been allowed by Vance. He would have made certain that there could be no mistakes.

Tom reported his findings and had the couples reconstructed. Shortly after, missile errors dropped to zero.

One week later while Tom was on the factory floor amongst the other engineers, a loud voice came over the speaker system demanding he report to the president's office. Everyone watched Tom as he looked up to the glass windows that overlooked the inside of the building. Tom shrugged and found his way to the office. In the president's office stood the president himself, as well as the military contracting officer.

"Dr. Law?" the president said, "How did you do it?"

Before Tom could answer, the officer interrupted and said, "Congratulations, Dr. Law. I just wanted to meet the person who did that study on the computer system. As a result of your work, we'll be buying it."

The personnel director was standing to the side and said, "I told you guys. He's a genius."

Tom stood dumbfounded, and after shaking everyone's hands, he returned to the factory floor. If only, he thought, it was always so simple as plugging in a few cables. Tom was pleased with himself, even though he didn't think his contribution was all that significant. He had promised the company a year, mostly because he felt he owed it to them for moving him out here. He felt vaguely guilty over that fact. Universities never went to such lengths.

Tom was pleased, but bored. Autonetics had been a fun experience for him and the company had rescued him from a difficult situation, yet there was not the same sense of discovery and adventure that he experienced in research. So during the few hours a week that he took away from work, Tom began to apply for research grants.

He had no idea what he would do with one if he received it, medical schools were obviously out of the question, but his mind still wandered back to the unanswered questions about the brain and behavior.

As he was emotionally recuperating during those first few months, Tom realized that his *real* work was incomplete, and he determined to find a way to finish it. He knew that he needed to continue to track the brain circuits that sequenced, programmed and executed reproductive behavior, not just the sexual behavior that typical biologists considered the whole of reproduction, but the various subtle supportive signals that comprised the entire process.

To Tom, this meant everything from initial attraction to courtship to the nurturing of the young. It was a foreign concept at the time in science, but Tom knew intuitively that for females, at least, so much more than just the act of sex itself was involved. He was determined to find the answers.

One day he was called and asked to meet with a psychological committee from public health services. After a lengthy discussion, the committee awarded Tom one million dollars if he would continue with his physiological research in neurology. Tom was elated and told them he would find a facility within a week, and he prepared to inform Autonetics that he would be leaving.

The president of Autonetics was gracious. "You didn't have to stay a whole year, Tom. What you did in the first six months was more than worth it to us. We're sad to see you go, but we understand. Congratulations on the grant."

Tom said goodbye and set about his search for a university that would accept him. Hopefully, he thought, the money he had been promised would help.

Chapter Nine

The young who never fear to die,
believe a chimera guards the closure of the day.

When Tom approached Claremont University with his proposal, their reception of him was ambiguous. Claremont was a small university that had gained notoriety for its graduate theological program. Much of the undergraduate curriculum was dedicated to preparing the students in liberal arts and philosophy, in anticipation of their interests in the seminary. The undergraduate science program was meager, and a graduate program in science was simply non-existent.

Both the president and the Dean at Claremont were uncertain, exactly, what to do with Tom, yet the possibility of building a graduate program, especially using someone else's money, was enticing. They were impressed with his credentials, yet they had little knowledge about his field. Most of what he explained about it left them thinking that Tom was some sort of psychologist, yet he was speaking about actually probing the brain and linking the 'circuits' he found there to behavior, reproductive behavior, in fact. It had never been something a theological university had concerned itself about, to say the least. Still, the committee from the public health services *must* have faith in him to offer such a generous grant, and they comforted their fears in light of that.

After some consideration, Tom was given a small space in a basement on a trial basis. He set to work immediately, building the first pieces of equipment that he would need from bits and scraps of lab materials that he scrounged from the chemistry and physics departments.

When the grant committee showed up to inspect Tom's facility, they examined his home-made cathode follower with its battery powered vacuum tubes suspended by rubber bands in a cardboard box and commented, "Well, we can certainly see you *need* the money…is this your shielded cage?"

"It works." Tom said. "I made one like it at Hopkins."

"What exactly will you be researching again?" They asked, then added, "Neural sequencing?"

"Yes," Tom replied, "I made a good start at it while at Hopkins, then more progress again when I taught at Michigan, but it was only a beginning. Most of the neural pathways are still unmapped. For that matter, neural secretion has never been studied, and while the whole of the scientific community knows and understands that the pituitary gland releases hormones that regulate our bodies, no one yet seems to consider what is actually controlling the pituitary gland. Yet the pituitary is right there under the hypothalamus. I've found some interesting things in the hypothalamus. More is happening there than we know."

The committee members raised their eyebrows and regarded Tom. Very few had any of his expertise in this field and he apparently had a knack for getting things accomplished, even when working with very little. The committee met with the president and the Dean that afternoon.

It was suggested that the school provide a larger facility for Dr. Law, and the president was quick to agree. "We could purchase a small building just adjacent to our campus," he said, as he considered the implications of having a million extra dollars in his budget,

"I'll see to it that Tom has what he needs."

The committee agreed, and said the funds would be made available within a week.

Tom was jubilant. The Dean had made it clear that Tom was to be teaching an inordinate amount of classes, including comparative behavior, neuroanatomy, neurophysiology, biochemistry, and biophysics. It would be overwhelming, but it would also give Tom the opportunity to find and recruit talent.

For the task that lay ahead in his ambitious dreams, Tom would need to surround himself with brilliance. The best students would stand out, and even if they lacked knowledge, he could train them. His plan was beginning to take shape. The foundation was laid. Now it was simply a matter of work.

The physics professor, Dr. Leonard Dart, was a Quaker, and one of the only two faculty members that appeared to be friendly to Tom. The rest, for some reason, seemed distant and aloof. Dr. Freeman Bovert, a chemistry professor, was also helpful in acquainting Tom with the campus and the administrative routine.

When it came time for Tom to outfit his new premises, Dr. Dart helped Tom acquire the equipment he needed, and what they could not buy directly, Dr. Dart had the skills to create. Before long, Tom had a lab that was rivaling his old labs at Michigan.

In the courses Tom taught there were some hopeful prospects for his project, but not enough. In his special graduate program there would be twelve students. They would be offered degrees in Physiological Psychology, which would be the first time it would be offered on this campus, and for that matter, possibly the world. Tom needed to accelerate his program, and to do that, he would need to recruit from outside.

Most of the faculty members disdained the administrative duties that encompassed sitting on committees, so Tom encountered little resistance when he offered to chair admissions. Once placed in that position, Tom started to see some hope.

There were applicants, he noticed, that never would have made it through the traditional admissions process. Housewives with liberal arts degrees or middle-aged workers that had a science background yet lacked credentials. Tom had worked with Nobel Prize winners and had learned to see beneath the surface. Most innovation, he discovered, seemed to generate out of misfits and rebels. Tom found and accepted an odd assortment of PhD candidates from the general population and proceeded to train them.

As his program developed, he gained momentum. The courses he taught were becoming so popular that students were in competition for his classes, and other faculty members either attempted to align themselves with Tom, or they spent their time and energy complaining to the administration that Tom was sequestering the best students and should relinquish some of his classes. The Dean, however, was overall pleased with the rapid and unexpected growth of the science department. There were enough funds left in Tom's grant money to build a two-story graduate science building.

Tom and Leonard Dart designed it, and when Tom moved his program into the top floor, Dr. Dart and the chemistry professor, Freeman Bovert, happily moved into the second story. The three worked together turning out top graduate science students that rivaled the credentials of long established universities.

At a certain point, Tom noticed that he had a team of first year students that were exemplary. It was time, he thought, to take his work to another level. The mapping of the brain, at least the portions he was most interested in, had been largely completed. Yet there was still the question of neurosecretion, and the scope of input into the reproductive center from other aspects of the brain.

It was time to put his students to work…

The small, brownish female rat blinked and sniffed as she was removed from her cage. She was used to being handled, so when Lauren reached in to scoop her up in his gloved hand, she only started slightly at the initial contact and made no attempt to bite him. Lauren caressed her briefly, and then placed her in the center of a large, low box.

At each of the four corners of this box were male rats tethered in such a way that they could freely move, but only about six inches from the corners.

Sophia, as this particular female rat was named, was in estrous. The male rats were acutely aware of this. They sniffed and pulled against their tethers, struggling to reach this nubile delight, as she coyly evaluated the situation from the center of the enclosure. Five graduate students stood around the box, clipboards and pens at the ready to record each and every action in this sequence.

It was Lauren's experiment. He was nearing graduation and while the university did not require publication to graduate, Dr. Law did. Laurens professor and mentor was clearly the most demanding of all the faculty members. Yet Lauren and the eleven other graduate students, or acolytes, if you listened to cynical comments from the faculty, would have followed Tom off a cliff.

Never before had their minds been opened to such a degree. Never before had so much been asked, and it surprised all of them when they were able to rise to his demands. Lauren had been there when Dr. Law cornered Kin Hiashi in his lab. Kin was Japanese and extremely talented, but he lacked incentive. Dr. Law had walked in on Kin one day while Kin was ignoring his work and writing a game program for the computer.

Dr. Law approached Kin and said, "You're not applying yourself. You're getting nothing done, and you're going nowhere."

Kin looked up at Tom and in a very apologetic tone said, "I'm so sorry, Dr. Law. I just have problem with the English. I have language barrier."

Dr. Law responded, in perfect *Japanese*, "You do NOT have a language barrier, you are just lazy!" Kins eyes shot up in surprise, and he immediately set to work.

That had been a year ago, Lauren reflected, and he had noticed that Kin, from that point on, was extremely productive.

The rest of them were similarly challenged in their own ways. Each of them had suffered unreasonable demands, but as a result, they had grown beyond their limits. They followed Tom without question.

The demand for publication was a serious one, and Lauren had approached Dr. Law with the concept for this experiment. There were many philosophical discussions that Tom engaged in with his students, as they commonly spent twelve, and sometimes sixteen hours together every day.

It was clear that Tom was setting out to prove something about reproductive behavior, something that went against the whole of the academic community. A great part of his work had been in physical, tangible proof. All twelve graduate students were now, as a result, accomplished surgeons. Some of them, Miriam LeGare for example, had so much talent that they could conduct brain surgeries that would rival top physicians.

Miriam had proved this recently when she made an astonishing discovery. She had located an optic nerve that had never been discovered before. What was unique about it was the fact that unlike the rest of the nerves that left the eye and traveled to the vision center of the brain, this stray fiber wandered along on its own until it ended, abruptly, in the hypothalamus. The research papers she had published, as a result, astonished the scientific world, and certainly pleased Dr. Law who, along with Miriam, concluded that this was even more validation that the hypothalamus was a central processing center. Miriam was smug in her accomplishment, but Lauren hoped to garner similar favor from their mentor via this current experiment.

Sophia moved a few paces towards one of the male rats. There was the sound of frantic scribbling on clipboards, and the creak of a chair as Dr. Law rose from his desk nearby to saunter over and observe the unfolding drama. There were high stakes on this love scene. All of academia was attached to the notion that the drama of reproduction in *all* animals centered on the choices that the *males* of each species made.

Males were stronger and in most species, males were larger. The world was filled with male scientists who all nodded in agreement that females were much like a row of fresh fruits on display at the local market. The male had but to go down the row and pick the finest one.

Dr. Law had one day voiced his disagreement over this. "Then why is it," he said to Lauren, "That the *male* peacock expends so much of his metabolic energy growing and displaying all that useless plumage? All those feathers do nothing to aid in flight, and if anything, they are a hindrance. No," he mused, "They could only serve the purpose of attracting a female. So you have to wonder just which gender it is that is on display."

"Wait a minute," Lauren had said, "Let's take a look at humans. It is the *female* humans that wear cosmetics, not the males." Miriam, who had been listening in, frowned at Lauren, but he ignored her.

"I agree," Tom said, "I'm certain that there is competition amongst both of the genders, and maybe that explains the cosmetics and maybe not. I'm sure even female peacocks have their standards to meet. But if we want to really know the answer, we should test it."

Lauren thought about it for some time, and then approached Dr. Law with his proposal. He would place a *male* rat in the center of an enclosure, and with estrous females around the periphery, they would see which one the male selected.

As a result of this experiment, they found two surprising things. The first was that every single male rat they used was more than willing to mate with virtually every single female. True, he had his first choice, followed by his second and third, but the fact remained that he would have all of them if he could.

"Typical," Miriam had commented, "Just like men...a bunch of pigs." But the second discovery in that experiment was more along the lines of validation. If an unpopular male rat were selected from the colony, the females would not mate with him. If he approached, they would simply sit down, effectively precluding any chance for him to have success.

Miriam nodded as she witnessed this. "At least female rats know what's right."

The second half of the experiment was the culmination of the premise, this time using a female rat surrounded by the tethered males.

Lauren stood waiting. Sophia was the center of his attention. Sophia made one complete circuit of the box, and delicately sniffed towards each male. She was making a decision.

There were four unique personalities represented by the four males. They had been profiled and categorized through countless hours of observation. Each graduate student, in his or her turn, had spent long sleepless nights and meticulously clicked off on a counter every action of dozens of male rats during courtship and mating. Courtship had been defined in three stages. The first was the initial contact, insignificant in the sense that rats made this type of gesture hundreds of times a day with every other rat they contacted.

The second stage showed more than casual interest. Noses touched delicately, and if compliant, the female would allow the male to investigate her body more fully. The final stage was brief but decisive. The female presented her genitalia and courtship abruptly ended with the beginning of mating.

Mating profiles were evaluated as a matter of duration and number of penetrations before completion. Male rats were then categorized into one of four personality types.

"Bashful" was very tentative in his approaches. Even when the female was willing, he was slow to approach and could easily be diverted to other activities, such as a sudden obsession with personal grooming. While the odds of success in a cage with an estrous female were nearly 100%, it was a wonder sometimes that Bashful ever got the job done.

"Sly" was a bit more assertive. He lacked the uncertainty of Bashful and made a more direct approach. If he were human and in a bar, the researchers anthropomorphized, he would tell the bartender to send a pretty girl a drink, and while she might accept it, he would probably chicken out when it came to sidling up beside her and asking for her name or phone number. Probably honest and forthright, Sly was a "regular guy" with good intentions. He held a steady job and was decent looking enough, however he came across as insecure. It was likely, the researchers postulated, that he drove a small Chevy.

"Gentleman Jim" was the next in the series. He drove a Corvette or a Porsche and had no problems with insecurity. He would not only send a pretty girl a drink at a bar, but he would send one to her date and have the bartender say it was from a different pretty girl across the room. By the time her date returned, all he would see would be the taillights of the Corvette in the distance. Gentleman Jim knew all the moves. Yet, he was mindful and aware. Advance too fast, and you get a sharp reprove. Too slow, and your time has run out. There were high hopes for this contender, and Lauren, whose very career was hanging in the balance, was nervous and anxious over Sophia's choice.

The final male rat profile was called simply "The Rapist." Direct to the point of aggression, he had only one thing in mind. Little attempt was made at courtship, since he was simply not into commitment. It was *all* about getting the job done. Granted, he was successful in rat colonies where there were no restrictions. He could, if there were no other males around to prevent it, mate repeatedly and with success, albeit often without consent, but in a social hierarchy, he was likely to be thwarted. It was postulated that there was some form of communication amongst the colony that garnered cooperation in preventing rapes, but which gender was in control of that was anyone's guess. At any rate, here was a situation in which there were no social restrictions. The female could choose whichever of the four males she wanted.

Sophia came close to Gentleman Jim and sniffed. She walked a few paces away and moved toward The Rapist. Lauren's eyebrows raised, then he frowned, but Sophia quickly veered away from The Rapist and moved back to Gentleman Jim. Noses touched and whiskers twitched, and soon there were the obvious signs of courtship. When the romance was in consummation, Lauren looked over at Tom who was smiling back at him.

"Good enough to publish?" Lauren asked.

"Good enough," Tom replied, "But repeat it a few more times with different personality profiles, just to make sure." Tom thought for a moment and then said, "Just so you are fully aware, when you publish this, you will become very unpopular. There are a lot of scientists whose reputations will become tarnished. Be sure that you are alright with that before you send it off."

"But will I get my degree?" Lauren asked hopefully.

"Yes," Tom said, "Finish your work here, and you're on your way. You'll have to take the orals, but they should be simple for you. I told you that if you publish and complete your course work, you would graduate. I'm really pleased for you, Lauren." Tom smiled. "You've worked hard and done a good job."

Lauren was jubilant and invited the rest of the graduate students out for the evening to celebrate. Over a pitcher of beer they happily discussed the nuances of social behavior, and started placing bets on which male in the bar would be selected for mating by the few single females. Lauren had placed a bet on a woman with large breasts. Kin had his money on a younger woman, who lacked the voluptuousness, but beat the other woman in terms of youth by several years.

"What *is* it with men and breasts?" Miriam asked.

"We don't have them," Kin answered flatly.

"No, seriously," she said, "*Why* the obsession?"

"Super releasers," Lauren said.

"Super what?" Miriam asked.

"Releasers," Lauren said and then continued, "Remember the experiment with seagull eggs? It was published a few months ago. I suspect this has something to do with that."

"I didn't read it," Miriam said.

"It was an experiment on the behaviors of seagulls that had to do with removing one of their eggs from the nest and seeing if they would retrieve it. As it turned out, they would always retrieve their egg."

"So what does that have to do with breasts?" Miriam asked.

"Well," Lauren continued, "They found that when they replaced the real egg with one that was larger, the seagull would go after the larger one every time."

"So you're saying," Miriam asked, "That there is a program in the minds of men that is similar to the program in seagulls, and that this program is based on the thought that 'more is better'. Is that it?"

"Probably," Lauren said, "At least that's what I think Dr. Law would say."

"Then why youth?" Miriam pressed, "Kin here has his dollar on the twenty-year old. If more is better, then why not more years?" Miriam was thirty-five and had two children. She resented the fact that men were inordinately attracted to younger women, and it seemed to her that as each year passed, she lost her social status in a subtle way.

"If more is better," Kin chimed in, "Then more children are better too."

Miriam looked at Kin. "Are you saying that the younger I am, the more children I can have and that's what attracts you?"

"Yes," Lauren interjected, "Look, if Dr. Law is right, then our basic programming is based on evolutionary advantage. If a male wants to pass his genes on to the next generation, then he needs to have children. If that male is attracted to a female reaching menopause, he is unlikely to have much success, so it's in his best interests to go after the young ones – children wise, that is."

"OK," Miriam said, "OK. Let's say that's true. But you, Lauren, just proved today that it's female selection that reigns. So why are males *allowed* the option? In fact, if we are following your premise and extrapolating it to humans, where are the peacock feathers? Where, in all of this, do you find validation that humans have a selection process that involves *female* selection? Frankly, I can see why the professors at Berkeley are going to rip you to shreds."

Lauren was momentarily taken aback. Then after a moment's thought he said, "I can answer that. First of all, in any given population there is competition amongst each gender. Larger breasts or youth on the one hand, more muscles or whatever on the other. While I would concede that a certain segment of the female population, those who are not able to reproduce, are not sought after by the males, for the remainder – for the females that *are* reproductively fertile, they are the one's who are driving the whole social structure. It's *they*, not the males, who are in control."

"OK," Miriam said, "Then show me some peacock feathers, Lauren."

"There," Lauren said, pointing out a window, "See that Mercedes convertible? The one with a forty-year old man in it? Do you really think that he wanted, suddenly, to drive around in the wind? Or do you concede that the expensive car, with all its impracticality and expense, is more or less a large set of antlers on an elk."

"Nice rack," Kin commented, and Miriam smiled.

"OK," Miriam said. "Let's just say that I'm going along with this," she started, but stopped when she noticed Dr. Law walking towards them.

"Mind if I join you?" Tom asked. "I don't want to interrupt," he finished politely.

"No. Please!" Lauren said, and Miriam scooted over to make room. "In fact, we were having a discussion about the experiment and maybe you can help."

Tom raised his eyebrows, and Miriam explained. "I'm not quite sure I understand this 'female selection' thing," she said, "If there were five women in this bar and one man walks in, it would be the *man* making a choice amongst the women, not the other way around, wouldn't it? I mean, isn't it just a matter of the situation and the options available?"

Tom contemplated a moment, then said, "Let's take a look at two potential examples. In the first, there are five men in the bar and a single woman walks in. What do you suppose she would do?"

"She would look the men over, I guess, and find out which one she wanted." Miriam smiled.

"Exactly," Tom said, "She would find out which *one* she wanted, and if this is to be a mating model, she would take that *one* home."

"All right," Miriam said, "But then what if there were five women in here and a single man walked in?"

Tom looked at Lauren and Kin. "Well," Tom said, "I believe it's most likely that the man would look the women over and certainly he would have his preferences, but if he felt he could get away with it, he would likely try to get them all to follow him home."

Lauren had been taking a drink of his beer and started to laugh, nearly spitting it out.

"It's true!" Kin said, "He might want them all!"

Miriam looked disgusted, but understood. She then said, "So when you say it is female 'selection' that reigns supreme, another way to say it is that females are the one's that are *selective*, and the difference is that men are less so or not at all."

"Yes," Tom said, "It's the example we see in harems."

"But why?" Miriam asked.

"Investment," Tom said, "The consequences of sex, at least prior to modern day birth control, are children. A man isn't making much of a sacrifice in terms of his investment. He's giving only a few sperm cells, and if he doesn't have anything to bind him to the woman, such as a marriage contract, then his donation to the process could conceivably be done. Yet the woman will be allocating huge resources. She will give much of her metabolic energy to the unborn child and because of that, she's bound to be selective."

"All right," Miriam said, "It makes sense from that perspective. But then the profiles of the rats in the experiment, how does she decide which one to mate with?"

"I can answer that one," Lauren said, "After all, this was my experiment."

Miriam waited, and Lauren continued, "If Sophia is going to have babies, and they are likely to be a combination of her genetic characteristics combined with the fathers, then she wants the babies to be the best possible rats around. In particular, if she has male babies, she wants them to be popular among the female rats when they grow up so that they'll have a chance at mating and her blood line will continue."

"All right," Miriam said, "Then if I understand you correctly, you're saying that Sophia ruled out the three personalities that she didn't like with the idea that if she had babies with them and they were little male rats, they would grow up like their fathers."

"Exactly!" Lauren said.

"But," Miriam continued, "If it's all about having numbers of children, why rule out the rapist? His sex drive is that of any other ten rats put together. Wouldn't that be all important in your model? He'd be sure to get the job done."

Tom was listening and smiling. He loved this sort of discussion, and it was wonderful to watch his students unravel the secrets and nuances of social structure.

Tom interjected, "Miriam, taking a human example for a moment, how did you select *your* husband?"

Miriam, momentarily taken back, thought about the question then answered, "I found a man who was attractive, kind and a good provider. One that I felt would stick around with me and help me raise my children."

"Does that answer your question?" Tom asked.

"I see," Miriam said, "The 'rapist' rat has plenty of drive, but no commitment. He wouldn't be likely to stick around long enough to protect the children, and as a result they might die and Sophia's lineage would stop.

"And," Tom continued, "What about the shy ones?"

"Not enough drive," Miriam said, "Their sons would not be likely to mate, and again she wouldn't have the continued blood line." Miriam smiled. "Good experiment, Lauren!"

"Why, thank you!" Lauren said back, smiling.

Miriam rose to leave. "Gentleman Jim awaits me at home," she said, "Good luck with your paper, Lauren." She bid them good night. Tom, Kin and Lauren waited a while, but left shortly after.

As far as the human experiment at the bar, Lauren and Kin were forced to call it a wash, as neither of their prospect women seemed to find anyone that evening.

Lauren was to take his oral exams two months later, and as the date approached, Tom became nervous. Laurens' paper had been published, and there were rumors that he may win the "Young Scientist Award" for his results. The award was given to the single best undergraduate scientist in the United States. So far, the new award had been given only once before and another of Tom's students had been a contender. The honor and acclaim this award levied was Olympic, and while it looked as though Lauren would receive it, there was the same old familiar dissention amongst the faculty at Claremont. Tom tried to pass it off as petty jealously, but it resurrected a similar feeling he had while at Michigan. Once the gossip mill started, he had found, the house of cards toppled rapidly. If it were limited to the faculty alone, Tom wouldn't have worried so much, but there was that incident with the Dean.

Tom and his students had been studying reproductive behavior for years, and that fact was well known at the university. While they tried not to advertise the details, the study of simple animals was limiting, and in order to take their studies further, they needed more. Humans were out. Tom had learned his lesson while at Michigan, but other animals had not been expressly forbidden. Earlier in that week the Dean had called Tom into his office. The nature of the call was unknown, but Tom was soon to find out.

When he walked into the office, the Dean exploded. "What the HELL, Tom!" the Dean said, "I took a site committee on a tour of your facility yesterday. You were gone, but we went by your lab."

"OK," Tom said, still completely in the dark over the meaning of this interview.

"Dogs, Tom! You have dogs up there in a locked room."

"Beagles," Tom offered.

"Dammit, Tom! They were screaming in pain! You could hear them three doors down! The committee was horrified. I was horrified. You're torturing animals up there! This will get back to the Regents, and so help me God, I don't know what to tell them…" the Dean's voice trailed off in despair. His look changed from rage to one of genuine anguish. His eyes had an almost pleading look as he waited for Tom to answer.

"Was this around four o'clock?" Tom asked.

"Yes, it was a few minutes before four, why?" the Dean said, still looking exasperated.

"Because at four o'clock every day, the estrous female beagles are released from their cages," Tom said, "We have beagles because they were at the pound and were going to be put to death. Their mating behaviors are being studied along with several other animals, and while beagles are ordinary dogs in every sense of the word, they do have a unique bray."

"Go on," the Dean said, although he was beginning to get the impression that he wouldn't like where this was going.

"Tell the committee that just as a beagle will bray loudly when on the scent of a hunting trail, they do so all the more when on the scent of an estrous female."

"I see," said the Dean flatly.

"The thing is," Tom went on, "The beagles bray loudly in ecstatic anticipation prior to mating, and the remarkable thing is they know when it is nearly four o'clock…the darned animals have actually learned to tell time."

There was a long pause as the Dean stared ahead at Tom. Slowly he collapsed in his chair like a deflated balloon. As he placed his face in his hands he muttered, "Dear God, I wish I had never asked."

When Tom left the office he knew that there would follow a growing dissention. How long, he wondered, would it take? Inevitably the prudery of culture would intervene, and like the postulates of Socrates, the administration would prefer to view the illusionary reflections on the cave wall rather than go outside and experience the light of truth.

It occupied his mind, and again he worried about the oral exams that were about to be given to Lauren.

If his sources were correct, the examining committee intended to fail Lauren, regardless of the fact that he was one of the brightest scientists in the nation. Tom had made a promise to Lauren, and he intended to keep it.

On the day of the exams, Lauren and Tom arrived at the chambers adjacent to the Deans' office. The head of every science department was present and sitting on one side of a long table opposite of which a chair had been placed.

"You're not required to be here, Dr. Law," the head of the psychology department said, "I'm sure you have other things to attend to."

"Not at all," Tom said amiably, "I should sit in on one of these now and then. Helps me to see that I'm doing my job."

The psychology professor regarded him silently, then continued, "Each department has one hour. You must answer every question, Mr. Gerbrandt."

With that, the examination began. It was evident from the beginning that they intended to fail Lauren. His knowledge of the material was vast, yet the questions asked were designed to have multiple correct answers, or they were so theoretical that the answer had no possibility of existing.

Tom's worst fears were realized, and he watched bitterly as Lauren struggled. Lauren made every effort. He had been prepared for everything except the hostility that faced him. Glancing nervously on occasion to Tom, he perspired and fought to maintain his composure.

Tom nodded reassuringly at Lauren when he glanced at him, then sat impassive as the barrage continued. By eleven-thirty the exam was only half over, and Tom interrupted, saying that his student needed a break. The faculty acquiesced, and while they murmured amongst themselves, Tom opened a bag he had brought with him and took out refreshments. Tom placed several chilled wine coolers on a counter, along with a large batch of fresh-baked brownies.

Lauren reached for one and Tom nudged him and shook his head with a short no, then said quietly, "I brought those for the professors." Lauren gave a puzzled look, but accepted the sandwich that Tom offered. The faculty spent some time with their own lunches, and as they finished off the last of the brownies and wine, the mood in the room lightened. A few of them asked Lauren about the award he was about to receive, and one actually shook his hand in congratulations.

When they settled back to the exam, the questions turned from stark animosity to open curiosity. "Why did you test the effects of hormones on hypothalamic cells?" one of them asked.

"Well," Lauren replied nervously as he glanced at Tom, "It was to see if homosexuality could be induced..." he trailed off.

"Could it?" asked another professor, who was fairly young and slight, and had been perceived by many as overly effeminate.

"Well, yes, actually," Lauren said with some enthusiasm, "We found that if there is a minor fluctuation in the estrogen balance in a pregnant rat, her male progeny will be homosexual."

The effeminate professor made some notes on his pad, then asked, "Do you think this could apply to humans?"

"It should," Lauren answered, "The hormones are the same."

"What about women?" a female professor asked, "Would this apply to them as well?"

"We never tested it," Lauren answered, "But by the same reasoning, it should. Neurosecretory balances in the limbic system are extremely delicate. Minor fluctuations can cause all sorts of changes in behavior." Several professors nodded and smiled. Lauren could not tell if they were mocking him or were genuinely interested, but at least the ambiance was no longer hostile.

Shortly after the exam was concluded, Tom left with Lauren.

"What in the *world*?" Lauren said to Tom, when they were some distance down the hall.

"They're high," Tom said.

"They're *what*!?" Lauren asked.

"T.H.C," Tom said, "I laced the brownies with pot."

"You did *what*?" Lauren said, as he stopped in his tracks.

"Shhh!" Tom said and then added in a hushed tone, "This is something you must not mention. Not to anyone. Ever."

"But they'll arrest me when they find out!" Lauren said in a loud whisper.

"Relax. They won't find out. None of them has ever smoked pot before and if they notice anything, they'll think it was the wine coolers. Besides, you saw how it was going in there. They were out to crucify you. I promised you would graduate and I keep my promises. By the way, I saw them grading your exams before we left. You passed."

Lauren stopped, unable to move another step and watched as Tom ambled on down the hall and turned to the doors that led out of the building.

He turned back toward Lauren and said with a smile, "Coming?"

"Hang on," Lauren said grinning, as he ran to catch up. The two of them walked silently back to the lab, where they found everyone had left for the day. There was a large balloon on Laurens desk that said 'Good Luck!' and it was signed by the eleven other graduate students.

The next day Dave French, another of Toms brightest, was the first to congratulate Lauren. Tom had been working with Dave on fertility studies and while Tom still felt squeamish over the past episodes with Dr. Behrman at Michigan, Dave was unlimited in his enthusiasm. The enthusiasm was contagious and eventually Tom allowed Dave to follow his interests.

"Congratulations on the orals," Dave said to Lauren, as he formally shook his hand. "I guess I have to call you Dr. Gerbrandt now," he added with a smile.

"Thanks," Lauren said, "But I still have to finish out the year."

"But at least the pressure's off now and maybe you can help me with *my* project," Dave said. Lauren smiled.

It was an interesting project to say the least. Some of the experimental psychologists had been testing biofeedback, and a good number of them were able to effect autonomic functions. Several of the grad students had been trained to lower the temperatures of a small spot on their foreheads, and the analyses that followed those results clogged the scientific journals. Dave, like the rest of Tom's group, was interested in the applications to reproduction, if any existed. Someone in Germany had suggested that sperm counts in human males were likely to be affected by temperature, in light of the fact that there was a rumor that the Japanese had traditionally, although with minimal success, attempted birth control via heating their scrotums in hot water. The thought was, that the high temperatures would kill a good number of the sperm. Dave surmised that if that were true, then the opposite might also prove valid, or in other words, cooling the scrotum might lead to increased sperm count and fertility.

Tom agreed that it seemed reasonable, yet his recent debacle over the mating beagles kept his enthusiasm down. It wasn't that he wasn't interested, it was just that he could see where this was going. Sooner or later one of his students would think of the obvious answer and when word got out, braying beagles would be the least of his problems.

It happened shortly after that someone, possibly Lauren, suggested to Dave that he conduct a study on the men in Scotland. Since they wore kilts, it should be a simple matter to evaluate their sperm count and compare it to the norm. Dave was excited, and after a brief investigation involving some cooperative physicians in Scotland, he found that the men who wore kilts did, indeed, have a slightly higher count. It was not long before an experiment was designed.

The male students and volunteers who had learned to reduce the temperatures on their foreheads were instructed to move the sensitive thermisters to their scrotums and continue with their biofeedback. Regular sperm counts had been taken before the experiment and they would be compared to the results that followed. Dave waited in anxious anticipation. After two weeks, the subjects were able to reduce testicular temperatures on a consistent basis and the first sperm samples were examined under microscopes to count and compare.

"Something's wrong," Dave said, as he peered into his phase contrast microscope.

"What is it?" Tom asked, and then sat down to look himself.

"There's hardly *any!*" both of them said in unison.

"Keep testing," Tom said, "It could be an artifact."

Dave tested every sample several times over the next few days, but the results were conclusive. The men were sterile. The experiment was immediately terminated, as Tom and the others worried that the effects could be permanent, but when the subjects discontinued with the biofeedback, their sperm counts returned to normal and everyone breathed a sigh of relief.

"This is huge," Dave said, "Regardless of the research results, there's a genuine application for this. Men could learn birth control and render all the clumsy apparatus obsolete!"

Tom agreed with Dave but was cautionary, "I would wait awhile before I let word of this get out, and I would run the tests again several times to make sure there are no deleterious side effects."

"I understand," Dave said, "But still. This is something that everyone can use."

Tom hated to squelch his spirit, but he had a premonition about how the university would accept this. The further from sea urchins and rats they went in their studies, the more infuriated the administration was likely to become. There was a recent flurry of discoveries his students had made and they ranged from the effects of pheromones on female dormitory students to the

161

multiple mating phenomenon they had seen in rats.

That last one made even Tom smile, as one of his group had nicknamed it the Coolidge Effect. A student had heard of the dialogue that happened between President Coolidge and his wife. It seemed that while the president was visiting a farm, his wife had made the observation that a rooster would mate several times in a short duration with several hens. When she expressed this to Calvin in amazement, he made the droll observation, "Yes, dear, but it was with several *different* hens."

Naturally, one of his students decided to test it and it held true. A male rat could mate several times with a single female before he was completely exhausted, but introduce a new female and he could start all over again. He could go on, far beyond his normal limits, as long as new females were introduced. It made sense from a social and biological standpoint, but it was another nail in the coffin lid that was closing on Tom's research. They all knew that the animals they were testing had behaviors that mirrored humans.

Sociologically, there was plenty of evidence that a human male would act similarly, as had been insinuated by the President, Calvin Coolidge. The social structure of the human culture did not take kindly to these observations and they were playing with fire.

The pheromone study had been another nail. Psychologists had made the observation that women, if kept in close quarters over a period of time, would begin to coordinate their ovulations. One of Tom's students had the bright notion to test it directly, and upon careful inquiry, found that freshmen entering into the woman's dormitory did, indeed, alter their cycles to a significant degree. It naturally followed, to his way of thinking, that there must be some biological purpose for this and testing was under way to see what effects males had on the olfactory senses of women.

A study involving subliminal armpit secretions in males and the effects they had on females was under way, and so far it appeared that women selected men to a high degree based on these factors.

It was hard to imagine anyone *not* being interested in these things, but then, university administrators were not scientists. They had wives and families, and a cultural and social structure that could not be understood by pure scientists.

But Tom understood. He knew that animal experiment mirrored human reproductive behavior, and that regardless of the arena in which the experiments were conducted, regardless of the pure and simple interests in furthering knowledge, the administration would draw the line. Dave would need to publish. Tom had made an edict that he would not bend, but aside from that, the results were of tremendous medical significance. Tom vowed silently that he would see it through, although he knew it would be rough for both himself and Dave.

One month later Dave was still working on the fertility experiment, although he had conclusive results and was fully ready to publish. He had found that there were no exceptions. It worked in 100% of the cases. He was in the process of pressuring Tom to let him publish, when Tom was called into the Deans' office.

The new chairman was there, Arthur Braifield, along with a face that Tom did not recognize. Tom was introduced to a new president of the university and then invited to sit down.

"You will not publish," Braifield said flatly.

"I beg your pardon?" Tom asked.

"These experiments on men's testicles, you will not publish them," Braifield said again.

Tom was irritated, even though he knew this was coming. "We will publish them," he said in defiance.

"You will *not*," Braifield emphasized and added, "If you attempt to, I'll see to it that you do not ever publish anything in the United States again."

Tom thought about it, and then thought about his career. He had thrown it away before, but he didn't relish the idea of starting all over again. Even if he had the energy, two strikes against him in academia would likely be his end. There were few, if any, universities that were not aware of him at this point. Too many publications, too many symposiums given and far too many cards stacked in the deck against him.

"Fine," he said, "I won't publish it in these United States." He then made a move to get up.

"There's more," Braifield said and Tom sat back down.

"We find that your performance is not up to our standards."

Tom was aghast. "How so?" he asked.

"Your students," Braifield continued, "They, by and large, leave your program and take menial jobs, such as teaching in state colleges. Your students are mediocre in every way and we at this university intend to turn out only high caliber professors."

Tom was infuriated and jumped out of his chair. He had expected to be criticized personally, but to attack his students was like piercing him in the heart.

He fought to control his anger and then said, "Let me get this straight, Mr. Braifield. The fact that my graduates are highly sought after in teaching positions in state colleges is *beneath* your standards? The fact that they have job offers prior to even graduating, which is highly unusual in this field does not meet with your expectations? How about the fact that two of the only three 'Young Scientist Awards' ever given are going to *my* students?" He continued, almost breathless now. "One of my graduates is now the head of a department at Dartmouth, another has an offer from the Max Plank Institute. Our research publications, from this tiny school, are higher in our field than any other California university and you have the *gall* to tell me that my students are substandard. Is that what I'm hearing?"

The faculty members rustled in their chairs and after a moment, Braifield said, "You're wasting your time, Dr. Law."

"You won't hear from me again," Tom said and walked out of the office.

Tom approached the faculty grievance committee, but while they were conciliatory, they were also completely ineffective. It was clear now that the new chairman and president had been hired for the sole purpose of eliminating Tom.

Tom explained his situation to his students who grieved as though they, themselves, were to blame.

"It's not your fault," Tom told them, "I knew the dangers and it was my mistake to bring you into this field. The world isn't ready for it and I'm not sure it ever will be." Then he added, "Dave, the editor of McGraw Hill is interested in your paper. We'll publish it in Germany. They can't stop that."

Dave hung his head and with the rest of the students sat in consternation over the loss of the greatest teacher they had ever known.

"Will you still speak at the symposium?" one of his students asked. There was an all-day lecture to be given by some of the top scientists in the world in one week, and Tom had been invited to speak along with two Nobel Prize winners. All of his students were excited to go and hear Tom lecture.

"Yes," Tom said and then thought for a moment, "Yes, I'll still go. Make sure you're all there. I plan to talk about what we have been working on."

Tom left the lab and his students and on the way out, he looked at his cherished equipment that he didn't expect to see again. There on the wall was the gas chromatograph and over there was the electrophoretic unit. The microscopes he smiled over. He was proficient now and he wondered if Dr.

Crosby was still teaching. He had finally mastered the use of them, and she would have been proud. With a final silent goodbye, Tom shut the door and walked home.

Chapter Ten

The worlds I made never passed by here,
Nor caught the bursar's grudging eye.
They lie vacant among the cinders,
Useless as the sand where
The corpses of the streaking stars
Lifeless lie.

Tom walked into the lecture hall at Northridge Lutheran and examined the audience. It was a fairly small group, as he had expected. There were, after all, two Nobel Prize winners who would be lecturing in the larger adjacent halls and in spite of all of his years in science, Tom was less well known. Also, he thought, it could have something to do with the title of his topic.

There had been a book published recently that was popular among the general public entitled *Sex And The Single Woman*. In a bold stroke Tom, at the last minute, entitled his speech, "Sex And The Single Cell." The word sex was still anathema among scientists, but at this point, Tom didn't care. He made a decision about many things in his life and was no longer in the mood to hold back.

Darren, one of Tom's students, ushered Tom to the lectern and checked the microphone. Everything was functioning well so, as the audience settled, Tom began.

"Honored colleagues, I have been asked to speak today on research. Specifically, research on the brain and the results we have garnered over the past two decades. But before I begin, I have to ask myself this question. Why did I choose the brain in the first place? The immediate answer, the one that I would have given years ago, is that there was so little known. I needed to find my niche in science, and as a physiologist, I could not rehash the old material. The brain was a new frontier and I admit that a large part of my decision was based on the selfish motive of creating a place for myself in the world.

That was the simple, partial answer, but in my heart I knew there was more. I knew that I had questions about myself, questions that have not and could not be answered by psychologists. To those of you who are in this field, forgive me for saying it, but personality profiles and subjective tests have never led me to a fundamental understanding of myself.

With all due respect to Freud and Jung, the science of psychology offers postulates that change and evolve over time. I am a physiologist. I need to know that what I believe to be true today will still remain so several years hence.

So, I built a probe and we examined the brain, cell by single cell. We started at the core, the hypothalamus, with the intention of working our way out from there.

Surprisingly, we found that we didn't need to; everything from the outer layers was, in some way, connected to the center. Just as the pressure you feel on your finger tips is nothing more than a signal that is transmitted to the central point, the brain, so the outer portions of the brain serve to communicate with its center, the hypothalamus.

To what end we ask? The answer is simple. Reproduction.

This statement may be disturbing to many, it *certainly* is disturbing to the administration where I teach, but the fact remains that without reproduction a species cannot exist. Why, I have asked myself, is this such a disturbing statement? Why do we fight so hard against it? Once again, the answer is simple. We have spent hundreds, if not thousands of years, in self-indulgent egotism. We congratulate ourselves for being so drastically superior to the rest of the species on the planet, that we center our theology on statements that "God" has given *us* this planet and all the creatures upon it. We are the center of God's attention. We are the special chosen ones. In order for us to feel secure with that thought, it is essential that we believe we are, in some way, qualitatively different from "animals." But much like the early astronomer who was placed in prison for suggesting that the universe did not evolve around the earth, we punish those who suggest that Homo Sapiens, man, our species is similar in fundamental respects to the other animals that walk, swim and fly the earth. In our ongoing attempts to define ourselves as unique, we take drastic measures to define other species as inferior. It's a kind of blue-collar deconstructionism. Our more verbal, but less thoughtful, spokesmen used to proudly claim that humans were the only creatures that could make tools and use them, yet we're finding that to be untrue. Chimpanzees and even birds are known to make and use tools.

We keep vainly searching for some trait that makes us distinct, the product of a personally concerned Creator, when, in fact, we should be *awed* by the intimate continuity humans have with all other life. It *is* remarkable that other species create tools, but memory and learning are *not* the peak of evolutionary accomplishment, as nearly every scientist claims. It is common.

All organisms learn and remember. We have evolved this wonderful large brain so we don't *have* to learn and remember so much.

So the question our fragile egos ask is, what is the essence of being 'human'? Why then this large brain? Before I give you *my* answer, I'll take the approach that others have taken. Their typical, pat answer is this thing we call consciousness. Yet that also, if we are to seek the truth about ourselves, requires a scientific investigation.

Dutifully then, we scientists investigate and ask the question; does consciousness define humanness? I would say, if I chose to think about it, that consciousness is a necessity, but not sufficient alone to define us. There is no 'human' without consciousness, but consciousness does not automatically confer humanness.

So maybe the problem lies in our definition, and maybe it's impossible to define exactly. But we can concede that probably just as with pornography, we will know it when we see it. We are pretty sure that higher primates are conscious. There is a plethora of documented behavior, such as deceit, planning, alliances and so on, which require consciousness; at least it does in us, and hence we infer its presence in them.

So now we have to grant that there is more than one member to this exclusive club, in other words, humans, chimps and for all we know, other species as well. This realization creates a continuum. There isn't a point of abrupt change and as a result, we see that *all* living things are connected, if any two species are.

Anyone who has ever owned a dog has no doubt in their minds that their cherished pet has a form of consciousness, but what about mice, rats or rodents in general? I have personally seen some behavior in rodents that would make consciousness hard to deny. It seems to spring from awareness on the level that we humans enjoy. Shall we drop to the level of birds with their very minimal brains? Deception in birds is well documented. So is planning in the form of storage, which presupposes the ability to project into the future. They also exhibit mapping, dialogue and altruism. Either we have to attribute consciousness to the display of these behaviors, or we have to redefine it and try to find reasons to disqualify the traits we formerly established as the indication of its presence.

As you probably guessed, there is no end to this revisionism of convenience.

So how far "down" do we go? We all too soon reach a point where the organism cannot demonstrate the traits we have selected simply *because* it hasn't the expressive morphology to do it. A worm can't wave to us without arms. We are reduced to searching for traits, which always accompany consciousness, even though they do not define it.

We have to be careful about relinquishing some of our favorites. For example, many theorists are fond of claiming the ability to recognize oneself in a mirror as a basic criterion of consciousness. How convenient. That pretty much keeps it limited to a high primate level, but we have begged the question, or in other words, the discovery is the definition. Animals then, who cannot look into a mirror or have no reason to, are disqualified, whether they are conscious or not. This eliminates the family dog, but not the family parakeet, which is problematic.

So then we say, one of the traits of consciousness must surely be learning! We have considered learning the highest function of the brain for decades, yet looking closely we quickly find that earthworms, cockroaches and flies learn. With a broad enough definition of learning, we find that even bacteria are capable. They have been observed to repeat motility into directions that lead to food sources and to 'learn' how to avoid noxious substances. How much farther would it be to question if indeed, consciousness might extend to the level of complex molecular organization, which pretty much comprises a bacterium?

It's not a far reach from that point to extrapolate to the level of DNA. If this is true, and I'm not necessarily saying that it is, then consciousness is, in actuality, a message.

It's the seeds of a blossom that become a lineage for billions of years. A message that's honed and polished over millennia, a message that is reborn each new generation and in the process, the information itself becomes changed.

We humans may not find that a particularly comforting thought, but for the rose, it's enough. We may find the fragrance of the rose ethereal, but that's a bonus only to us. To the rose, it's only important that the fragrance is a beacon to honey bees and pollinators that says "here I am." The rose doesn't give a damn that it smells good to us, that's irrelevant to the design of its fragrance. It cares that it is cocaine to butterflies.

We are like this rose. We keep trumpeting, in endless ways, the message "here I am" in a sense advertising our link to life. How we do this is by virtue of our brain.

Then what of consciousness? How would our definition change if we accepted this as truth? We would likely surmise that it increases the chances of having more offspring for ourselves than our competitors have. We would start to think of consciousness as a scanning device – it monitors all the senses and their perceptions and in turn focuses and organizes the data from the senses. The process provides an integrated evaluation of perceptual data, its significance, its survival urgency and ultimately its value. It's not such a far reach; since judgment, evaluation, prediction and relation are qualities we traditionally attribute to consciousness.

The validation of all these factors came from the study of the brain, the reaches within which we found all the systems that support these functions. We discovered, and it should not be surprising, that there is a place where all of the inputs converge. Logically there *has* to be such a place.

There must to be a place that controls the release of hormones related to stimulation, to smells, to predator threats and the environment. It must be a place that receives the inputs from all of the emotional systems and it must, in order to be effective, be close to the neurosecretory cells.

When our probes found the hypothalamus, we knew that we had located this central processing center. Create a lesion here and you have a female rat that will not go into estrous. Create one there and you have a nymphomaniac. Change the sounds, the lighting or the emotions of the animal and you cause changes in the cellular activities of the hypothalamus.

Now, the question we asked ourselves was why all the extra gray matter in our *human* brains? The hypothalamus is ancient in the evolutionary scheme. It has been there from the time of reptiles. So what is all the extra brain matter for?

Before I answer, reconsider the continuum of consciousness. and the fact that human genetic material is only a fraction of a percentage different than that of chimpanzees. That small percent may give us an advantage, but looking over our social structure and comparing it to that of chimps leads us to ask some pointed questions.

Our minds encompass, retain, employ and manipulate our world, as well as its people and its resources. We derive the wherewithal to increase our numbers exponentially from a small genetic advantage. But does that signify an increase in the qualities of our new brain vs. one with which we made flint knives or herded elephants over a cliff to harvest them?

Long ago we could carry seeds across a desert from one climate to another. But that, along with other ancient technologies led to the same results as they do today, the increases in technology serve primarily to increase our population. We are able to have more children, and we are able to live longer.

Have we made a qualitative difference in our minds over the minds of inequity? How much closer are we to cooperative living on an inclusive basis the whole of the species, instead of local groups? The monkeys and chimps are as far along in that as we are and no farther. Have we any new ideals? Do we underwrite those we claim to have? Are we feeding the world, allowing free dissemination of information? Have we made old age productive and rewarding for our senior citizens?

Medical treatment is about as advanced from the theory of humors as technology is from obsidian tools, but how much closer to universal availability is it? How far along is representative government? We govern ourselves as the baboons do, by allies and relatives. Of all these things we pretty much accept in a consensus, all the desirable improvements in society, and child rearing, and city planning, and planet engineering and resource conservation, yet, through it all, how much have we actually *done*.

No, the increase in our brain size has yet to exhibit a significant, fundamental, qualitative difference. We are the same as our kindred – the other various and wonderful species that inhabit this planet. We are more complex, but like them, our basic motives are simple. We reproduce."

Tom paused in his speaking. He realized that for the past several minutes, he had not been following his notes or outline. In fact, he couldn't remember just how far back he had diverged onto this philosophical track. He had been thinking out loud, in essence, and with a wry inward smile he realized that these musings were, by and large, a reflection of his personal frustration over the limitations of humanity.

He looked up at the audience and noticed that the room had filled considerably. The room was absolutely silent, yet full, and people trailed into the halls.

Darren, Tom's student, caught Tom's attention, and motioned him away from the microphone. "We have to move you," Darren said.

"I'm about to get lynched, aren't I?" Tom said.

"No," Darren said, "There's not enough room in this hall. They want to move you into a larger one."

"Oh," said Tom.

Darren made an announcement that the speaker would take a thirty-minute break, and the group would be moving to auditorium C.

Tom followed Darren, and over a small lunch they made polite conversation for several minutes. When it was time, Darren ushered Tom into the adjacent lecture hall and once again, checked the microphone. The hall, although considerably larger then the prior one, was completely filled.

Tom cleared his throat and looked up. He wasn't sure where to begin.

He had made some deeply cynical remarks that, while he considered them to be true, were far off the mark in terms of physiology. Yet, he thought, scientists are humans too. They have families and friends and live in a world of relationships. When they leave the biochemistry lab, they walk the streets like any other person and smile at a handsome man or flirt with a pretty girl. They pay taxes and have political opinions. They have a personal religion or they make a point to not have one, but behind it all, beneath the surface, they are just as human as a jazz singer in a nightclub or a professional athlete. We all question the meaning of life, Tom thought.

He began again, attempting to find where he had left off.

"Somewhere, around four or five billion years ago, a rather uncomplicated molecule underwent a remarkable change and duplicated itself. At that same moment, new meaning entered into the universe.

Meaning is not an intrinsic quality. The equation $a = b + c$ has no meaning. It is nothing more than ink spots on paper. To a nonmathematical reader it is an incomprehensible use of three letters of the alphabet. They spell nothing, therefore they mean nothing.

To a mind with only a smattering of arithmetical education, it's a sum and totally meaningful. The arithmetical mind has been educated and primed with a linguistic social convention. If you put 'c' potatoes in the basket and you put 'b' potatoes in the same basket, then you will have a basket of 'a' potatoes as a result.

The instruction of the operation to be performed has resulted in the ascription of meaning to the symbols, which represent, but do not explain, the operation. The meaning is there when the operation is done. The meaning is *not* there when the operation is absent.

Please, let's not waste time on 'emergent' qualities. I place that in the category of 'phlogiston' and 'the ether' and 'quintessential' elements. Nobody ever saw one and nobody can imagine a way that one could.

By the same reasoning the molecule that replaced itself did not possess the meaning of duplication. The event came about because of a unique combination of forces and the matter they acted on. And the same thing would happen again whenever the instructions for combination were carried. The *meaning* is in the *operation*.

To extrapolate, the meaning of the sum, is in the procedure used to arrive at it. The meaning of reproduction is in the operation and the machinery necessary to bring it about.

If things, which reproduce by themselves, are living things, then the meaning of living is in the operation of life or reproduction without entropy.

Therefore, the meaning of life, ladies and gentlemen, *is in the living of it.*

We have taken a grand journey into the depths of the brain and unveiled the secrets there. Perhaps, we were like Columbus and thought we would be discovering India, but what we found, though not what we expected, was even more exciting. The intrinsic drive to reproduce, to procreate, to find our lover and take him or her to bed is the 'new land' and yet, we discover it has been there for eons.

Still, like the puritans of our early American history, we find it distasteful. But why? It's a program that was written and perfected over millions of years, and it's beautiful in its completeness. We don't have to obey the programming. We can become conscious of it, and in our awareness, we can choose to take whatever direction we want. We may decide to become monks, nuns or to abstain in any number of ways. We can live in self-denial or hedonistic self-indulgence. We are free to make the choice, but the freedom is not won by ignoring the truth. The brain has a program that is inherent and hard-wired, and all the connective machinery has been designed to support it. All the hormones, all the sensory inputs, all the subliminal suggestions of our higher mind belie this fact. Whatever you may chose to do with this information, whatever course of action you take, you will feel the influences.

Your brain, to distill it down to the most basic essence, is by and large, a sophisticated reproductive organ."

Tom finished with that final statement and picked up his notes and walked out of the lecture hall. Behind him there was a stunned silence. One thing is for certain, he thought, Claremont would not be welcoming him back.

He said a brief goodbye to his students who were waiting for him just outside. Their faces were beaming and they let him pass as he gently pushed by them.

In the parking lot he paused and looked back. His students had followed him out and were standing a few paces away. Tom mounted his motorcycle, on which he had packed his few possessions – some camping supplies and one or two books that he could not bear to part with.

"Good luck," he said to them, and he started the motorcycle and rode out of the parking lot, heading north.

One week later, Tom contacted Darren who had left messages at several campgrounds. Tom was concerned that there was an emergency, but when he heard Darren's voice he was reassured.

"You missed it," Darren said.

"I know," Tom said, "I still value my life – that's why I left."

"No!" Darren laughed, "You missed the party! You should have seen it; they nearly brought the house down! After you left, people broke up into small groups and lots of them ended up at my house. Someone suggested we verify your experiments. So picture this, a group of scientists sitting in my living room with their pants off, trying to cool their testicles."

"Oh my," Tom said. Then after a moment's pondering asked, "How did you manage to measure the temperatures?"

"That's the best part!" Darren said, "The women were holding them to check."

"But…" Tom started, "That would actually raise….ohhhhhh. Never mind….." he trailed off.

Tom was chuckling as he hung up the receiver. He turned and walked back to his small campfire by the ocean where he was preparing to roast a fish he had caught that day. He had placed the fish on a rack made of small sticks and bailing wire. He sat on a board held up by two stones holding his homemade roaster and smiled to himself as he stared into the flickering campfire.

Chapter Eleven

Lost in the wind strong grove of shimmering blooms,
Petals trembling with laughter in the sea breeze,
I touched with delight –
Barely restrained –
The yellow trumpets of joy
and plucked just one.

It was a wounded and sorry soul that pulled into the parking area late that day. His Honda motorcycle was muddy and so was he. They both looked to be about the same, depressed and bedraggled, ill kept and showing signs of too much wear and tear. Tom got off his Honda, stretched his saddle sore body and looked around. It was a beautiful area. Plenty of pine trees covering the rolling hills with lots of streams and wild flowers in this month of late May. It gave him the feeling of being very deep in the woods, but in actuality, it was the terrain that made it so, as it really wasn't that far off the beaten track. All the better, Tom thought to himself.

Esalen Institute is tucked snuggly among the big pine and eucalyptus trees of the Big Sur area that is located in the steep hills of the Central Coast of California. The ocean is so close that the waves can easily be heard from Highway 1 as it meanders along the steep terrain. The whole area is noted far and wide for its beauty. It was also noted for paying a reasonable amount of homage to the hippy movement, some of whom drifted down from San Francisco. They also found it a beautiful place to be while exploring their hallucinogenic, drug-induced sojourns. The resident property owners had little use for the liberal drug movement, but stuck it out for the sake of the incomparable beauty.

Tom didn't know what to expect at Esalen. He had only vaguely heard about it in off handed comments from his associates. It was reputed to be a place where individuals congregated, "daring in their thrust for understanding and knowledge and thus, ultimately, defining and embracing the eventual acceptance of one's own self," as the brochures read. Tom had decided to head this way. He had dared all right. He had dared the entire scientific world, and they had not only accepted his challenge, they had made it perfectly clear that he was beaten. The intellectual life had betrayed him, he realized. He had lost everything, his career, his professorship, his wife and children, his home and all his money. A life of study and dedication and devotion to students – all of it didn't matter any longer. The powers that existed, the powers that had ultimate control, had assassinated him. They had demanded his loyalty, yet cared little of his dedication to facts and scientific epistemology and had wantonly tossed him into the cesspool and walked away. It seemed to him, that the 'straight' world had nothing to offer. It had betrayed him, and he owed nothing to them in return. He owed nothing to Truth and Beauty.

He considered his plight and decided that a true scientist was always willing to offer himself to the opposite or 'null' hypothesis. What if one considered these possibilities? What if, for example, magic is real and works at a distance? What if there is truth to spirituality and all the precepts of religion? Forget, he thought, the torch of light that scientists burned. Theirs is a myopic blinder that belies their prejudices. It's time to look to the opposition for a change.

Tom carried with him the clothes on his back and some camping gear. There was little else. None of his papers survived. None of the awards he had won in his years of teaching. No plaques, ribbons or written acclaims. He had left it all behind, so deep was his disappointment and feelings of rejection.

So here, at Esalen, he thought maybe he could find his answers. They were reputed to have an "open arms" policy, and he intended to put that policy to the test.

As he pulled his motorcycle into a parking space, an attendant came to greet him. "Welcome!" the young man of about twenty-five said, "Are you attending a seminar?"

"Not exactly," Tom said, "I'm looking for work."

"Oh." The face fell on the attendant. He hesitated, then said, "You can try in maintenance, they may need someone there."

Tom asked for directions and then made his way to the maintenance building. He walked through the doorway and discovered a young man, probably about twenty-five, hunched over a video tape player. There were pieces of the broken machine all over the table and the man was cursing at it.

Tom looked at the components and then cleared his throat, startling the repairman. Before he could speak, Tom said, "I can probably help with that."

"It's busted," the man said, "I don't think it is fixable."

Tom smiled and poked at the components. "The transformer is burned out," Tom said, "I can make one if you have a volt meter." The man handed Tom the meter and watched in fascination as Tom found some wire, wound it and tested it several times. After a while Tom had the machine back together.

"What seminar are you attending?" Sean, the young man, asked.

"I'm not attending," Tom said, "I'm looking for work."

Sean took a deep breath and sighed, "Well, it's clear we need some help with things around here, but besides running the video equipment we really need just general maintenance, like gardening and heavy labor stuff." Sean was eyeing Tom, who did not seem particularly fit and certainly was a good deal too old for real work.

"I'll take it," Tom said, "I can use a shovel."

Sean cleared it with the administrator, and he was hired.

Tom worked in general maintenance for a month, sweating in the afternoons over walkways that needed repairs, and mending fences and door locks. When he was finished for the day, he was allowed to attend seminars. He found them fascinating. Everything they taught went against his background. Guru's sat with students in meditation and, on occasion, chanted. Tom joined in with alacrity. He had closed off the scientific portion of his mind and left it behind. Now, all was openness to this new reality. He sat and listened and joined in with the diverse array of broken hearts and troubled minds taking refuge at Esalen. There were divorcees, grieving parents, and those who just wanted a place to heal and to find a different way of life. A life that might afford them a change from all the hurt they were experiencing.

The courses were interesting, and the instructors even more so. Tom was particularly interested in one Guru. He was reputedly one of the nation's best and he was the inventor of a process whereby the students could learn to reconstruct their lives using a large box filled with sand. The box contained various artifacts, and the student was to climb inside and rearrange the items into a perfect order. Each item was meant to represent a significant part of their life. When it was Tom's turn, he climbed in and stacked a bunch of stones in the corner and buried them under the sand. The rest of the box he smoothed out, turning it into a gently flowing Zen-like pattern. The group watched with interest, and when he was finished, the Guru asked Tom what the stones had represented.

"A bunch of old crap in my life that I don't need anymore." Tom told him. The Guru smiled and gave an approving nod to Tom, then went on to explain to the rest of the group how Tom was one who "got it." Tom was pleased, but really, deep inside, he could not imagine that burying the stones solved anything about his past. It was just a fun exercise to him, and these people were finding significance that apparently escaped him.

After a few months Tom began to notice a change in the way these particular people treated him. Many times, he was approached and asked for advice. Tom shared freely with everyone, and with his past in teaching, even began to take on some of those attributes. More and more, it seemed, his role was changing. Over the course of several months the demands from the maintenance crew lightened and he was asked to assist in seminars. As his role changed, Tom reflected on the types of people he was teaching. He had no way of knowing just how much his inherent and distinctive qualities would relate to the masses of people in this completely different environment, but he gave of himself and as a result was greatly appreciated.

In particular, he was viewed as a healer. His background in Medical Schools facilitated an understanding far beyond the typical instructors. Tom would participate in holistic healing with guided imagery. The laying on of hands often worked. One woman in particular improved over time with such drastic changes that Tom became her savior. Tom struggled with the situation, partly because the adoration was embarrassing and partly because his scientific mind could not accept the process, in spite of the fact it was working.

Despite his reservations, Tom acquiesced to help the endless stream of hurt souls that flowed through Esalen. He devised a series of guided images that helped take the individuals through their pains and ultimately wrote an outline of techniques. The staff watched in appreciation as their erstwhile maintenance employee began to draw his own crowd. Unbeknownst to Tom, plans were being made around him. Behind his back and without his knowledge, he was being touted not just as a learned Guru, but there were hushed whispers of his being a true Shaman.

Shamans were the ultimate draw in those days and their workshops brought in the most money at Esalen.

Tom was soon approached by a noted Guru and cordially invited to attend a small, but 'world-wide' gathering at a clandestine hilltop somewhere in a concealed area in Mexico. He was told it would be a wonderful, "once in a lifetime" experience and that this particular gathering happened only once every ten years. It was only open, they told him, to a select few and there would be many Shamans from all over the world.

Yet the greatest draw was that one, very special Head Shaman would attend. Tom agreed to go, feeling that this was possibly a very special honor. The trip was carefully planned and thought out. Timing was of utmost importance as was complete secrecy....not a word was to be mentioned to anyone, especially at Esalen. No family members were to be told; even the time they were to leave was to be kept from the general knowledge of everyone.

When the secret day finally arrived, they took a small bag of toiletries and silently met in a prearranged place away from the eyes of the other people at the Institute. The buses were parked around a corner from the actual parking lot and were not readily in view of the public. They drove in a caravan of three in VW buses. All together, there were about 16 people including Tom and the Guru with his companion.

The trip was laborious and miserable and took about a week, with the usual troubles of flat tires and engine problems. Tom was enthusiastic at first, but began to have reservations when they arrived in Mexico. They had driven endlessly over poor roads throughout the night. Only the main driver in the first bus seemed to know where they were going and he refused to share that information. Tom's apprehension grew. It concerned him that of the entire group, he was seemingly the only one concerned that their destination was being concealed. He looked nervously over the gathering of people and his mind became analytical about the whole situation.

Here, he thought to himself, was a group of true followers, not leaders. Leaders would care where they were going and certainly why. Followers were all too ready to be herded like cattle. Tom focused his attention on the roads in an attempt to calculate their location, but it was dark and the roads were unmarked.

Finally, the bus jolted to a stop, and they were instructed to get out. Tom considered attempting to turn back, perhaps leave with the driver, but the group ushered him up along a narrow trail - it was clear that they had specific intentions. They walked for what seemed like miles up a hill and over a rickety wooden bridge, and after about three hours, they came to the top of a mountain. Perched on the highest point of the mountain were several large buildings outlined eerily in the night sky.

By now the moon was out and they could see the silhouette of the main building. It was large and appeared to have a bell tower, and Tom thought it might have been an old Monastery. It looked grayish and crumbling in the moonlight as it perched precariously on a flat area but seemed to be surrounded with sand.

A tall, slender man in a robe, who gave the impression of being especially interested in Tom, greeted them. He bent over to look into Tom's face, but his breath smelled of stale wine and garlic, making Tom turn involuntarily away. The man, nonplussed, led them into one of the buildings and they walked down a large hall with open arched windows. They were then each assigned to a small room that contained nothing more than a cot and a wooden dresser. There were no windows, but the rounded wooden door had a slider about one foot in diameter that opened from the inside only. Tom felt a sense of growing panic. It seemed more like a prison cell to him than a hotel. He calmed his nerves, however, as he reassured himself that this was, after all, to be the experience of a lifetime, and they were soon to meet and have access to several world-famous Shamans.

At about 5 am the next morning they all assembled outside their rooms and were led in file to the dining hall. The drab surroundings complemented the prison-cell rooms, but after several questions were asked and answered, they were told there was a shower and they could clean up. The shower, they were to find, was heated by a wood fire, but wood was scarce and as such only about three of them had hot water. The bathrooms were meager and dirty and while the food was good, Tom's mood became darker.

By the third day, Tom had spoken with several Shamans. He visited with them as they sat around and spoke softly in small groupings, but it disturbed him that the conversations always seemed to be directed toward him. Tom was adept in every field, from philosophy to medicine and even massage and holistic healing; yet it was strange to him that he saw some recognizable symptoms in this group. They acted as though they were the students and he was the teacher - Tom easily recognized the signs from his years as a professor.

Fortunately, the big event that they were all waiting for was drawing close and Tom's attention turned to the coming event.

The Head Shaman was about to make his presence known and the postulated outcome was that there would be many "teachings and healings".

The excitement grew for all of them and Tom felt partially caught up in it. Here was one who was the Shaman of all Shamans – the one who would greet them with high wrought, pure emotion, which would compel them into Shaman-type actions. Yet in spite of this anticipation, Tom began to notice that everywhere he went there were people with *him*. They followed him, and while he didn't think much of it at first – after all they barely knew one another – it started to feel…different. For one thing, Tom overheard several people commenting on how much money they had spent in getting here, yet Tom himself had been charged nothing. He couldn't understand why the others had been required to pay.

There were conversations that the others had, often in Spanish, and Tom, unbeknownst to them, understood the language enough to make out most of the meaning. He caught glimpses of an emotional undercurrent that unsettled him, and his apprehension grew.

There *had* been many workshops focused on mysticism and healing, so time was passing quickly. Yet *besides* that, Tom noticed that he was never, ever alone. To an increasing degree people were around him asking questions, and then…some of them began to touch him. At first he thought it was just because they felt they knew each other, but soon it became obvious it was more than that.

One morning he came out of his room to find five or six young men on the floor with expressions of reverence on their faces sitting at his feet. He almost tripped over them. Their actions were excessive and he suffered a bag of mixed emotions over the situation. He assumed they were misguided because the Head Shaman hadn't shown up yet and they needed an older figure to guide them. But he was embarrassed and later when several of the women did the same thing. It began to scare him out of his wits.

They had all been given robes to wear while there, and then one or two of the worshipers began to hang onto the bottom of his robe as he tried to walk. They would let go when he pulled on his robe, but the whole thing was too much for Tom.

In desperation, he found the Guru who had enticed him into coming to the place and asked him when the Head Shaman was coming, thinking that at least once he knew, he could spread the word and get some of the heat off of himself. He mentioned to the Guru that things seemed to be getting a little out of hand, but the Guru just looked at Tom and smiled, and said, "Tom, don't you understand by now? When all the Shamans are congregated in this place, they secretly vote to elect the Head Shaman, and… it's you! You are the chosen one!"

Tom was stunned and his mind raced. He couldn't believe what he was hearing! No wonder, he thought to himself, all of these people were constantly following him. It flashed across his mind that some of them would be very disappointed with what they probably paid to see and experience – that being a real, honest to goodness, Spiritual Shaman.

His next immediate thought was escape. He had no means of transportation; in fact, he didn't even know *where* in Mexico he was. He thought furiously and then it all began to fall into place. Everyone had thought *he* was the Head Shaman all along – everyone, that is, except for him and his stomach which was turning over and getting ready to heave up it's contents. His body lurched in a swaying unsteadiness.

What if, he thought, they decided to lynch him? Especially when they realized they'd paid good money and he wasn't what they thought he was supposed to be? Here he was, a kindly, short and aging Professor who had a few extra pounds on him, graying at the temples and not in particularly good shape. Could he outrun them he thought? No, he reasoned, not most of them. He desperately tried to think of how to handle the situation. His imagination envisioned him running as fast as his short, little legs could take him down the road followed by an angry horde of betrayed followers. He pictured himself flying down the God forsaken road, clearing that wooden bridge towards the bottom like a Kentucky racehorse, followed by a screaming, machete-wielding crowd closing in on him. He could just picture it. Tearing along, gasping for breath, wondering if anyone would ever find his mutilated body.

He controlled his imagination, which had obviously gotten away from him for a second, and tried to think rationally. There was one thing he wholeheartedly understood and that was that he had to get away as quickly as possible.

Gathering his thoughts, he made the announcement to everyone that he had a case of "the tourista" and would need to stay in his cell the rest of that day. After dinner, he hurriedly returned to his room, making excuses to all the worried faces that had stared at nothing but him throughout the entire meal. He decided that he could not get out of there fast enough, so he gathered his meager items into a small knapsack that he had brought with him. As soon as it was dark he slipped outside into the sparsely wooded area. When no one was looking, he ran. He ran like he had never run before in his life. It had taken them three hours to get up, but it only took him one hour to make it down. He longed, in between gasping thoughts, for his old Honda motorcycle, but he was traveling almost as fast without it.

When he reached the road, he didn't know which way to go, so he picked a direction and struck out. He walked the rest of the entire night, and when it was just getting light, a speeding truck, apparently hell bent for election, squealed to a stop and picked him up. He was saved.

It took Tom several days to wind his way back to the border, and he had never been so thankful to see anything in his life as the border station and its beautiful American flag waving in the breeze. As soon as he was near a phone, he called a friend and begged for a ride home. It was over, and he had suffered a narrow escape.

On the long drive back into central California, he told his story to Richard, a friend whom Tom had know at Autonetics. Richard said little, since Tom could not stop talking. He had to tell someone about it, mostly to make sure that he was not imagining the whole incident. When he was finished, he mused about the adventure and admitted that he would never really be sure whether or not he was actually in serious trouble, but that being said, he remembered the look – that subtle, darting movement in everyone's eyes and felt that his instincts to run had been well served.

Tom fell asleep and Richard drove straight through to Morro Bay on the central coast of California and dropped him off. Tom had sailed into Morro Bay a time or two while living in southern California and teaching at Claremont and had a good feeling about the small fishing port. Richard let Tom out of the car, told him to stay in touch and headed back to southern California. Tom stared after Richard's car until it was out of sight and then walked towards the waterfront, found a bar and ordered a pitcher of beer. He watched as the sea birds wheeled and screeched in the afternoon sun and reveled over the fact that for the second time, he was running from serious trouble.

Chapter Twelve

On the carved edge of the sky, one lone brown silvered mote,
Stonefall of ragged bird, rushes down the shallow day
To jar the solid sea.

Tom met Rennie while he was living on a little 14ft. houseboat in Morro Bay after he left Esalen and returned from his sojourn in Mexico. He was finished with Esalen. He had learned all there was to learn about that alternate way of life and he considered it over. However, he didn't really quite know what to do with himself at this point. He felt betrayed by both ends of the spectrum, and there seemed to be nothing that he could get excited about in the interval that would help him establish a balance in his life.

When he wandered into Morro Bay, he decided it was as good a spot as any to throw out his anchor and rest for a while. It was a peaceful little fishing village, and people tended to live and let live for the most part. Tom found it healing, and the solitude he enjoyed while fishing and crabbing restored his heavy soul and slowly he began to feel some of his enthusiasm for life returning. It was easy to reflect back on his early manhood days in West Virginia and his corncrib cabin in the mountains. That had been a healing time in his life as well, and it amazed even him that his life had taken so many odd turns since those days so many years ago.

Now he was alone once again, on a boat and a long way from his boyhood home in West Virginia.

Tom sometimes felt an overwhelming sadness. It came and went like the tide and eel grass, but it was there, lurking in the background all of the time and ready to thrust its head up and glare at the sun soaked sky of Morro Bay. "Why?" Tom wondered to himself, "Are things really that bad now?" After all, he was still alive and in good shape physically. And then slowly he realized, it was over. His life long career of discovery and published papers and teaching; the excitement and thrill of the improbable discoveries, the soirées, the great talks, the swapping of ideas and outlooks, the metamorphosis of a consensus of ideas, all of it, over. There wouldn't be the motivation of the great minds of antiquity, Plato, Aesculapius, Aristotle on his little houseboat. No, the presentation of inspirations and the scrubbing of them in the common bath of constructive criticism were over now. He was...*retired* and he never meant to be. Why, he wondered, was just the mere fact of being retired, never mind all the rest that was just quotidian honey gathering anyway, such a mental blow? He was far from the improbable undoable Aegean stable task of expanding his mind. But now he must deal with the fact that a major door in his life was closed forever and the closing had been anything but pleasant or satisfying. It would take some doing and certainly some time, to open another door and it would be harder still to walk on through.

While surrounded by people at Esalen he hadn't really dealt with the finality of it all. Hadn't had time. Now, alone at last with time to heal, he laid it out on the table, turned it every way possible and eventually, as was his way, prepared to deal with it.

He found the little houseboat, moved onboard and lived on $50.00 a month poaching oysters and crabs and fish that he caught in the day and ate at night. Perched precariously on the stern of his boat sat a little barbecue which served him well, and between that and the oriental market which was within walking distance of the harbor, he managed nicely.

Tom enjoyed being anchored out in the bay. There was no direct access to the boat so one had to stow a skiff on shore and row back and forth, but it was quiet and private. He soon became used to waking up to the various sounds of the different kinds of sea birds. The graceful, white Egrets made raucous squawking sounds when nesting in the tall eucalyptus trees that lined the shore – and admittedly, that took some adjusting - but all in all, the beauty of the bay and its natural inhabitants provided a peaceful serenity. Tom found the time alone to be valuable for his much needed healing. For company, he had the gulls and the otters. On occasion a seal would poke its head up next to him and they would silently regard one another. Neither of them said anything, but something passed between them nonetheless. Tom would throw scraps of fish out, and the seal would disappear, perhaps finding the morsel or perhaps just leaving – he was never sure which.

Tom began his slow climb back into the world, and after a time, he began to feel lonely. When on the boat, his contact with people was minimal. Only the occasional fisherman would venture by, but they only waved and never stopped. Tom waved back and returned to the maintenance of the houseboat or his fishing, yet eventually he discovered he was ready to be with people again. In light of all that had happened in the past he took this as a good sign.

He began to linger around the marina a little more and was willing to meet and talk to others. He still had a few old contacts and occasionally he invited visitors out to the boat. He would make a point of inviting a new person each time, so that when they were having a barbecued dinner on deck, watching the sunset and the reflections on the water, he would be broadening his circle. There were professors that would gather. They would discuss philosophy and the political nature of academics, but Tom rarely joined in on these conversations. He smiled and nodded in understanding, but he didn't want to bring up his past. He was still too tender. It was over and sometimes all but forgotten, but still it brought instant pain back to his heart to think about it.

Tom was open to everyone and as a result some of the friends he gathered were misfits like him. Devout motorcyclists gravitated to Tom and forgave him for his academic brilliance. He was growing a beard and living off the land. It was all the confirmation they needed in order to feel comfortable.

He found and purchased an old motorcycle and began to ride again. His biker gang led him to reclusive areas and they would camp out at night, drinking wine and exchanging stories. Tom felt as at home with them as he did with professors, and it amused him to think of the various roles he had played in life. There were few women as yet that Tom encountered, but he had met one girl that attracted him. She was short and slightly heavy, but she had bright eyes and a contagious laugh. Tom found her extremely desirable, but try as he might, he could not get her to visit him on his houseboat. It was frustrating and he felt insecure about himself.

One night, he accepted an invitation to ride to the neighboring town of Atascadero and join his biker friends at a bar. Tom lamented his romantic woes to his friends, but by the time he was fully into his self-pity, most of them were fully drunk and not overly sympathetic. Tom drank along with them and was thinking that he had best pull himself out of his dark mood, when *she* showed up at the bar. She was with a male companion and made it clear by ignoring Tom that she felt she was far better off with this new friend. Tom was disgusted and offended by her actions and decided to leave in a hurry. He knew that he had been drinking too much, and normally he would have eaten something, but this evening he threw caution to the wind and with reckless abandon he mounted his motorcycle and left for home.

The road back to Morro Bay from Atascadero is two lanes and winds in and out of the coastal mountain range for several miles. Ordinarily, it is perfectly suited for the Honda, so Tom decided to push his speed to the limit. It was a foolish mistake, and the last thing Tom remembered was a curve with a large rock that loomed immediately larger – and then nothing.

Tom was stunned when he woke up in the hospital the next morning. He soon discovered that not only was he alive, but as a result of his foolishness, he had thirteen broken ribs and very little skin left in several places on his body. He was encased in a cast, from which only his legs and his right arm protruded. He hurt from his head to the bottom of his feet. In spite of being grateful to be alive, he realized that it would be some time before he could move normally, if ever. He berated himself for his stupidity. It was one thing to lament over a lost love, but this was an action suitable for a teenager.

Tom's friends visited him that day in the hospital and they brought him gifts, one of which was a small stick that he could maneuver down the cast to scratch the inevitable itches he would be experiencing over the next several months. They joked and laughed, and Tom's spirits lifted somewhat, but after they were gone, he suffered a revelation. His houseboat was anchored in the middle of the bay and there was absolutely no way he would be able to row out to it. He thought about it while lying in bed, but could come up with nothing by way of a solution.

He found that he would have plenty of time to think about it since he wouldn't be released from the hospital for quite awhile, but still, at the end when he was released, nothing presented itself. There was one possibility, but it came to an impasse. If he could move the houseboat to a dock, he could easily manage. The only problem was that the Dock Master had assured him that there was a ten-year waiting list and that houseboats were not really allowed permanent dock space regardless.

Tom tried originally when he was first there to convince the Dock Master of his obvious needs, but the only comment he would make was, "Sorry. Impossible."

Now Tom had real, critical reasons to be at the dock, but he doubted the space was available. Even if there were a space, the Dock Master would never let him have it after all the things he had said when Tom had first talked to him.

He deliberated over these thoughts and eventually gave up thinking about it since he couldn't find any answer. He would just have to find a way to survive when he was released.

Three days later Tom was standing outside at the marina looking towards the water and his boat. A friend had given him a lift back to Morro Bay from the hospital in San Luis Obispo and now, uneasy on his crutches and in pain, Tom had ambled down to the water to contemplate his situation. It was grim, he realized. There was not a single space available anywhere on the docks.

Dejected and disgusted he had just turned to walk down to the Dock Masters when he heard an unmistakable roar in the background. It grew louder and louder until he saw several Harley Davidson motorcycles pull into the parking area and stop right beside him. His friends slowly parked their bikes, grinned at Tom, dismounted and walked up to him. They gathered around him, and joked about his pathetic appearance, attempting to get Tom to react, but when he explained his situation they stopped. They quietly exchanged words among themselves and after some discussion they seemed to arrive at a decision.

As if in a well-performed ballet, they remounted their bikes simultaneously and turned towards the Harbor Master's office. Tom couldn't see the office clearly from where he was standing, and he noticed that several of the men, in full leathers and carrying chains, walked into the office and remained there for several minutes.

Within a matter of, what seemed like seconds, they walked out, turned toward him and waved. Then they rode the short distance back and gave him the news.

"It seems," said the spokesman for the group, "That we were somehow able to find you a space at the dock." The man gave Tom a wink, and then several of them launched Tom's skiff and rowed it out to the houseboat. By the time they had retrieved the boat, the Dock Master had found Tom and apologized profusely for not noticing that there was a perfectly good space available. Tom shook his head and thanked the Dock Master. Then he thanked his friends, who had saved him albeit through questionable methods, and hobbled down the dock and climbed aboard his boat. It was sad, he thought, that politics was such a rough game, but it was good to for once, to be on the winning side.

Tom healed slowly over the next several months. His fishing had to support him now, as crabs were harder to catch inside the slip area, but he rarely went without food. As he healed, he grew bored again. He was still missing companionship and challenge, so when a professor he was acquainted with offered him a job teaching, he readily accepted it. Tom agreed to teach, but only on the condition that it would not be science and the professor, who was conversant with Tom's background, agreed and understood exactly why.

He told Tom that what he wanted to teach would be his choice, yet he was frankly surprised when Tom announced that his subject would be massage. This was to be an experimental college, so there was great latitude in the curriculum, but to have a notable scientist teaching massage was a novelty. However, they agreed to allow it and Tom made preparations for his first class.

Among Tom's newest friends was a young couple. The husband was a sailor and rode sometimes in the biker group. His wife was a free-spirited young woman with long red hair that reached down to her hips. Tom knew from the early sign-ups that his class would be nearly full, with over forty people signed up already, and more possibly on the way. He was nervous, not because of the fact that he had never actually taught massage, but for the fact that people were so often squeamish about their bodies. Tom had learned to let that go at Esalen. In those days, the human form was openly displayed there in unabashed nudity. He realized that the conservative group signing up would need an event to break the ice, so he enlisted the aid of his new friends. Miriam, the redhead, was to be a 'plant' in the first class. She enthusiastically accepted the role of waiting until Tom was lecturing on the inherent beauty of the human body, and upon the pre-arranged phrase inviting a volunteer from the audience to come to the table, she was to boldly take her clothes off completely and come forth. It was meant to be a joke, of sorts, and at the same time, it would break the tension and the ice. Tom anticipated that this action might well alienate several class members, but at the same time, it would be a test as to their commitment at the beginning.

On the fateful day, the class congregated in the room and Tom readied himself. Marian was waiting in the audience and when Tom uttered the key phrase, she began to unbutton the top of her blouse. Yet much to Tom's amazement, there was another woman who was faster. Tom watched in fascination, as a tall, stately woman with long flowing hair calmly dropped her robe to her feet, exposing her nude body and smiling, silently walked up to the table. Their eyes met and held for a moment and then the woman laid down on the table and relaxed. Tom stood shocked and speechless for a moment, and then quickly glanced up to Marian who was smiling and rebuttoning her blouse.

The woman on the table looked up at Tom and smiled again. "I'm Rennie," she said.

Tom gazed back, mesmerized, and after he could compose himself said, "I'm Tom."

"I know," she said.

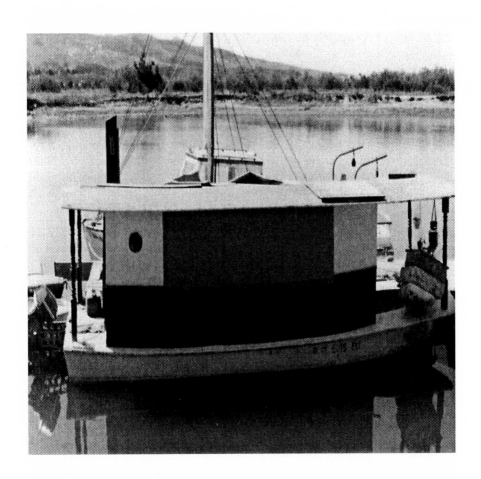

Chapter Thirteen

"A smile that blazes still"

Reinnette Clark Law was born in Ohio on September 21, 1915 to Mr. and Mrs. Edward Ford Clark. As the eldest of three children in one of the wealthiest families in the world, she grew accustomed to the diverse but interrelated kind of life and living that only the privileged enjoy. Yet for all the opulence, she did not, in fact, derive much satisfaction from all the physical things her parents provided. Her siblings didn't suffer similar frustrations, as they readily embraced the power and control they exerted on the servants and other people around them. Even at an early age of life, her younger sister, Elizabeth, was extremely fond of making the lives of the servants miserable in every way she could. "Joshua!" standing with her hands on her tiny hips and mimicking her mother, she would say to the butler, "How many times do I have to tell you that the kitchen floor has a stain on it?"

Joshua would stand straight, apologize and promise to see to the correction immediately, yet as Reinnette watched from the adjacent alcove, she knew that the stain, if ever there was one, would most likely be a streak in the pattern of the expensive marble tiles. Elizabeth would smile in condescension, and Joshua would do what all the employees did, bow courteously to the wielder of power and move hastily so as to satisfy his mistress. When he walked by Reniette, a glance would be exchanged; it was a look of compassion and acceptance that was rare in this household.

All of the employees knew that Reinnette was unusual. She had been coddled and trained just as the rest, yet for some strange reason, she was unspoiled. Even though educated in private schools, the ones that specifically exist to create a form of aristocratic nobility and garner an attitude of superiority, Reinnette could be found in the stable helping feed the horses and chatting openly with the stable hands. It was a source of conflict in the household, as Reinnette had been forbidden to fraternize on numerous occasions.

A schism was growing that mirrored the fundamental difference in attitudes between the aristocracy and the common working people. Reinnette threw her hat in amongst the masses. She protected them and fought for them, and her family tried desperately to convert her to their way of thinking. All to no avail.

A crisis was reached when Reinnette's eighteenth birthday was approaching. She had ventured one day to a small nearby airport and immediately fell in love with the thought of flying. This would be so much better, she thought, than jumping her thoroughbred Arabian, something that had been forbidden and an action that brought great disapproval from her riding coach. This would be flying! The feeling she had in the air riding her horse was over in seconds. This, she thought, would be that same feeling, yet sustained for minutes or even hours.

As her birthday approached, she was calculating and cautious. It would require some careful manipulation to get her father to agree to flying lessons, and her mother would never approve. Yet, there was always a way.

Two weeks before her birthday, when the family was assembled in the formal dining room and the silver serving dishes had all been placed by the host of servants, Jonathan Warner Clark II, Reinnette's father, broke the silence following the evening prayer. "Reinnette, have you decided what you want for your birthday yet? Before you answer, I have to tell you that there is a villa in France that's not far from Paris. I have good contacts and information about it, and it's yours if you want it."

The table was silent as the family looked at Reinnette, and she glanced at her mother before answering. "I think that's a most generous gift, father, but my home is here and I want to be close to my family."

"Perhaps a house in town nearby then?" her father asked, "You need to own property, dear. You need to show your young suitors that your family supports you or the best prospects will go elsewhere."

"Father," Reinnette began carefully, "Everyone already knows that we're wealthy. It's not a matter of my owning personal property that attracts suitors. If anything, they're intimidated by it."

Her younger sister snorted in derision, then said, "It doesn't hurt, and you know it. The more you have, the more they want you."

Reinnette ignored the remark and returned to the question of her birthday present. "If, father, I were to ask for something unusual yet something that I want more than anything in the world, could I have it?"

In a rare moment of generosity, Jonathan Warner answered, "It's your eighteenth birthday. Name it and it's yours."

"Flying lessons. I want to take flying lessons."

"No!" Reinnette's mother blurted out and then shot an angry glance at her husband.

"Typical," Elizabeth remarked, but she closed her mouth when her mother gave her an angry glance as well.

Her father was silent for several minutes as he gazed at his rebellious daughter. He seemed to be calculating the circumstances and weighing out the costs verses the possible benefits. At length, he responded, "If I allow you to take flying lessons, then you must agree to accept the husband I choose for you. Given, of course, that he is suitable and obviously from a good family."

Now it was Reinnette's turn to contemplate, as this was a negotiation that she should have seen coming, yet she had missed the obvious. On the one hand, she was elated that her dream of flying could be realized, yet on the other hand her father had a breeding program intended for her that was designed to keep the family wealth and image well protected. It was deplorable, she thought, to acquiesce to *anyone* choosing your husband for you, yet regardless of her becoming a pilot, the family plan for her would remain the same. She was educated, but not for the sake of a career. She was being groomed to be an aristocratic wife. The quiet, respectful, high cheek boned, frail and needy wife that men of power sought desperately to have. Given that road, she would become the quiet wife in public and at social occasions, and the bitter and unfulfilled woman in private – the type of woman that her mother had become. It was not a thought that she could tolerate.

Her father was waiting for her answer, and she gave it. "Yes, father, I agree, but only after I finish with my flying lessons will I be ready for your suitors."

Her mother smiled and seemed pleased, and the issue was decided.

Two weeks later Reinnette found a flight instructor and began her lessons. She quietly listened as Richard, the young instructor, explained the basics of aviation and the operating controls of the small two seat trainer.

Within an hour, she was in the air as the fabric winged craft lifted off the dirt runway. Richard glanced nervously at Reinnette as the plane lurched hard in a sudden air pocket, but she was calm and alert, so much so in fact, that he had her take the controls after only a few minutes in the air. He had expected this high-brow to quit in the first ten minutes. In fact, he had barely checked the weather as he figured it would be one lap around the airfield and he would be depositing her back by her car, as green in the face as the field she was parked on. But instead, she grasped the controls and turned confidently right as she applied the correct amount of rudder and then neutralized the ailerons. She was a natural, if ever he had seen one.

When they landed, Reinnette joyously climbed out and asked when the next lesson would be. The aviation business was slow, and Richard needed the money, so they agreed to meet every day at 9:00 am. Thanking him, Reinnette gave him a shy smile and turned and left.

On the third day, Richard crossed his arms and refused to touch the controls. "You can do this, Reinnette, give it full power and trim for take off. It'll fly off the runway when it's ready, don't rush it." Reinnette was nervous, but kept her wits about her. There was a slight cross wind on the airfield, so the right wing dipped as they lifted off, but she corrected with left aileron and remembered to keep some pressure on the right rudder. Richard smiled and said nothing.

"Where are we going?" Reinnette asked over the engine noise.

"Climb to pattern altitude, then turn back for landing."

"You'll take the controls then?" she asked.

"No," he said, "You're going to land us. Watch your airspeed and if we fall short of the runway just add power." He smiled at her and her heart did a little flip-flop, but she didn't have time to think about it.

Reinnette added flaps as she turned her base leg, then rounded out and lined up the runway. It appeared to be growing fast in the windscreen and she fought the temptation to pull up on the yoke. At fifteen feet she cut power and held the nose level until she felt the ground effect. She started to drift, but stepped harder on the rudder to correct, and just before contact with the ground, she pulled back and held the nose off until, at last, the plane bumped onto the dirt and taxied lazily down the runway.

Richard was beaming. "Perfect!" he yelled.

Reinnette was perspiring but exhilarated. "Let's do that again!" she exclaimed.

"OK. Twice more and then you're on your own."

Following two more 'touch and go's,' Richard debarked on the edge of the runway and turning to Reinnette, said, "You're a complete natural. Just do exactly what you have been doing. I'll be waiting right here. Don't worry. I wouldn't send you up if I didn't know you're ready."

Reinnette swallowed hard, then turned the plane to taxi back to the end of the runway. She felt a bit of panic as she lifted off and turned right – the airfield was small and the air was becoming bumpy. She felt terribly alone and wondered for a moment if her family was right about living a normal, conservative life. But as she turned back and circled towards the runway for her landing, she knew that her life could never be lived in stodgy mansions, ordering servants around and planning for the next evening affair designed to impress boring people. She leveled off on her final approach and added power. There was a head wind now, and she would fall short if she kept the engine at low RPM's. Her landing was textbook and she gave a scream of delight as she turned towards Richard. Jumping out of the plane, she ran up to him and embraced him. They were both laughing and Reinnette felt a tug in her heart. It seemed to be a mixture of the love she had for flying and a strange new feeling that was centered on this man. They laughed and held each other for much longer than was proper, and then Reinnette pulled away and confessed to Richard that she thought she could be falling in love with him. Richard flashed a quick smile, and then became serious.

"I feel the same way about you, Reinnette, but I have to tell you, business is slow here and I'm thinking of leaving. I think there's more opportunity in California, and I have an offer to run a flight school out there." Reinnette's face fell and Richard continued, "I know your family. They would never allow this. You...we...are not in the same league. I would take you, but..."

Reinnette cut him off, "I want to go. I have to leave anyway or my father will arrange a marriage for me, a marriage that I don't want." She looked away and then Richard reached out for her and pulled her close.

She had tears running down her face, and he brushed them away and whispered, "OK. It's settled then, we go together."

It took Reinnette a full month to gain the courage to tell her family that she was leaving. Mr. Clark exploded in fury, and seeing the rebellion in his daughter's eyes, stormed from the room and refused to speak to her again. Mrs. Clark was quietly furious, but determined. "You will listen to me, Reinnette," she said, "You don't know a thing about the world. Do you think this world welcomes the poor? Do you think that the life we live and the things we have come easily? There are more failures in life than successes, and even our family has had its share of disappointments. Here, I want you to promise you'll read something. These are the writings of your grandfather, Dr. Samuel Mathews. He too left for California during the Gold Rush of those days, and he ended up living a miserable life searching for his fortune. I want you to read these letters. We've saved them to remind us at times like this just how good we have it here." She flung a bundle of parchment on Reinnette's lap and stormed out of the sitting room.

Reinnette watched her mother leave, then stared down at the papers. She had heard a little about her grandfather, but the family was much more inclined to talk about the "successful" side, the side of the family that had entered the steel industry, and thanks to the bombing of the steel mills in Germany during the war, had inadvertently become one of the worlds leading providers.

Reinnette untied the bundle and the roll fell open in her lap. She began with the first letter.

> March 30, 1849
> Dear Huldah:
> As the steamboat has lain by a few hours this morning on account of the dense fog, I improve the opportunity to begin a letter, for when the boat is in motion, the jarring of the machinery makes it almost impossible to write legibly. We are on a good boat, the Captain a gentleman, and the waiters very attentive. I intended to write you by Alfred but finding so excellent a boat then all ready to start, and only waiting with the hope of concluding a bargain with us, we were obliged to pay our drivers and hurry on board.
> I walked about 10 miles each day, feet got sore, dropped my thick boots and tried the thin ones, but found them pretty thick, greased them, walked ten miles into Beaver without socks on, but my feet continued sore. This is a sure way of making them tough.
> One of the hands of the boat was drowned from falling overboard in getting off one of our wagon wheels. It was extreme carelessness. He was standing on the tariff rail or edge of the lower deck some two feet above the water, and the wheel was almost on the edge of the boat, so that when he pulled the wheel off - coming easier than he supposed, he fell in and the wheel after him. We have lost the wheel, but suppose the boat is liable, as we have a receipt for the Co. passage and three wagons.
> As the boat is getting up steam, I must close soon. We shall get to Cincinnati tonight, and lie there tomorrow.

I shall probably write you from St. Louis or Independence.

Yours respectfully and Affectionately,
Sam'l Mathews

Missouri River, Friday eve, April 6, 1849

My Dear Huldah,

We are now on the Missouri about 40 miles above its mouth, on board the S. Boat Mandan, Capt. Beers. We left St. Louis this morning at ten. We ran on a sand bar; it was too near dark to admit sailing any more tonight. A storm has been pouring for an hour or more, and it is quite refreshing, after a hot day. The scenery has been rather tame.

We have purchased everything except the animals and have money left sufficient to buy either oxen or mules with a nice balance in the treasury.

Every thing is harmony in the company.

The storm has passed off, the Moon is shining and the boat is about to proceed. So I must wind up as it is impossible to write when in motion.

I bought in Cincinnati a very heavy pair of blankets, napped on both sides for $4.50 and we bought in St. Louis a good Buffalo robe apiece for about $2.50.

From the crowd going over, it is impossible almost for us to have trouble with Indians. We shall not start from the frontier before the 1st of May. However, our time will not be wasted. We have some fixing to do on our tents, wagon - everything for so long a journey needs to be loaded very carefully so as to avoid friction and economize room.

Kit Carson will not lead any of the Companies, as he is beyond the mountains.

Col. Bryant of Louisville, Ky., is now at St Joseph and will probably take in charge the expedition from there. He is an experienced traveler in the far west, California, Mexico, and Oregon.

Tell me whether you are now reconciled to my absence.

There are five or six gamblers aboard, some of who played all night last night and have been at it all day today.

The Co. are all in excellent spirits. My old dress coat goes well, as it has been quite warm. I have had to wash my hands 3 or 4 times a day to keep decent. There are no ladies aboard, and I am in the ladies cabin quite comfortably located. There is some good scenery on the river but none very grand.

Yours affectionately,
S. Mathews

Fort Laramie, Tuesday, June 5 1849

My Dear Huldah,

I am hearty, have got tanned, wear nothing around my neck, and eat 3 times a day, have been cook one week, drive teams and close cattle frequently, walk 15 to 20 miles a day with some fatigue which is diminishing, have $18.00 dollars left and am resolutely bent for California as when I started and more so.

I suppose, notwithstanding I have left you for so long a time and gone on such a journey, you are still and will be anxious to hear from me. We heard horrible stories of Indians ahead but when we got along to them found them to be bugbears, built on the misfortunes of imprudent and extravagant travelers.

I have not shaved for a month but wash occasionally. I have no more time and must bid you adieu. I send you a pressed flower I have carried for several weeks in my book.
S.M.

From Huldah to Dr. Mathews
East Cleveland, July 4, 1849

My Dear Husband:

I do not know of any way that I can spend this day better or more agreeably than in writing to you. I have received three letters from you since you left home; one from Cincinnati, from Jefferson City and one from St. Joseph, dated April 20th in which you said that you should certainly write me once more before you left that place, but I have not received that letter or heard from you since.

There have been various reports in circulation about the Painesville Co., one that they had disbanded on account of the Cholera and were on their way home, and as I heard nothing from you I thought perhaps it might be true and that you intended to surprise me by making your appearance here.

But my hopes were soon blasted, for in looking over the Cleveland paper last week, I saw a notice of the death of Mr. Adams of the Painesville Co. It seems that he died of inflammation of the bowels 150 miles from St. Joseph. From this I conclude that you, if living, are really on your way to California.

I think that Mr. Adams' death must have been a heavy stroke to you as well as his relatives here, but we cannot stay the hand of death, however eager our pursuit after Honor, Wealth or Pleasure. How little he thought when he left home that he would be so soon summoned to Eternity. Truly we know not what a day or hour may bring forth.

I have just received a letter from Mrs. John Mathews saying that C. Adams had received a letter from you dated Fort Kearney May 14th giving an account of Mr. Adams death. It was received at Painesville July 2; although it is nearly two months since it was written, it is quite a relief to me to hear so directly from you, for we had a report here that you and all of the company but four were dead. Perhaps you will think me rather weak minded to be troubled on account of such reports but we have worse accounts than this reported that are found to be true. One company of 25 all died but 5;

200

another of 30 and only one survived; many similar cases.

Have you had any cases of cholera? Is it as bad as reported? Mrs. Mathews says that you were 300 miles from St. Joseph when you wrote. If so, I am in hopes that you have escaped, for the newspapers say that they do not have it that distance from the settlements, but perhaps they do by this time.

If you receive this I wish that you would tell me all you know about it. What would I give today to know that you are alive and well and getting along well with plenty of food for yourselves and the animals.

We rather wonder here at your going with oxen rather than mules. Every ox team I see reminds me of you, plodding your way along over prairies and mountains. I think that it must be dull, tedious business, not lonesome, however, for I should think that you would be as much annoyed with company as you were on the steamboat, from the accounts that we have of the number going over. So you find your expedition as agreeable as you anticipated? Do you not sometimes wish yourself at home? When do you think of returning? How do your funds hold out? Have you enough to make yourself comfortable in such an expensive country?

The cholera is prevailing considerable about here. Over 100 cases in Cincinnati for several days in succession; as many at St. Louis, some though not as much in the Eastern Cities. It is just commencing in Cleveland.

Your affectionate wife,
H. Mathews

East Cleveland, Sept. 25, 1849

Dear Husband;

This is the 5th anniversary of our marriage. Have you thought of it today? Or are you so much engrossed in your cares and pursuits that you have neither time nor inclination for such reflections? And now we are separated thousands of miles apart, perhaps never more to meet. All seems gloomy and desolate, but there is one consolation at all times, an all wise Providence reigns and if it is for the best we shall be permitted to meet again and enjoy each other's society and a quiet home.

I want you to write two letters to my one, not because I think mine are worth more than yours, but of course, I feel more anxious to hear from you than you do me. I am comfortable with friends and you are in a strange country where it is predicted there will be much suffering this winter.

Your affectionate wife and well wisher.

H.O. Mathews

Yuba River, Sunday, Dec. 16, 1849

Dear Wife,

Your two letters postmarked July 7th and August 22nd I read a few days since at Vernon, our nearest P.O. about 40 miles distant, to which place we had ordered all our letters forwarded from San Francisco.

We have provision for the whole winter for three of us. There is quite a settlement where we are, perhaps 150 to 200 men, 1 or 2 families, and all of them provisioned. The Sabbath is well observed as it would be by the same persons at home, especially if they were in one place. I know but little of the people on the bar but I hear no noise indicating a row or quarrel. I have not heard a fight or murder so this is quiet and safe a country as the world can exhibit.

My health is good, and I have often thought that I am stronger, tougher, longer-winded & healthy every way, soul, mind and body and estate. There has not been a case of Cholera in the country.

I practiced medicine for awhile after getting here, and occasionally on the route in the Co. and out of it. I have doctored every member of the Co. since our arrival. $5 a visit in the Co. $8 or $10 any distance out of it. It is no profit, but only an accommodation. The time and hindrance to a mess are great objections to practicing in the mines.

How do I like the country? Tolerably well! "Rather cool!"

Have I any intention of settling here? Now, Wife, that's where you got me. Do you suppose I have formed any intentions on the subject? Do you suppose I am bound to tell you my intentions, if I have any? Don't you suppose I would if I were bound to? Don't you suppose I see, even at this distance, what the object might have been in asking such a question? Now, before I answer your question, answer mine, and satisfy me whether, if I had answered yours in the affirmative, you would not have immediately applied for a Bill of Divorce, and used my letter as testimony against me. Therefore, in view of all these things and others that might be mentioned, all I will say is that until I get a larger pile than I have now, I have no intention of settling in any country.

Yours affectionately,

S. Mathews

PS. Last winter, as the Parks' say, the snow fell only twice, and they worked almost every day through the winter. The father and mother returned to the States in the Spring with over $30,000, leaving 3 sons on a good claim working Indians, to get another pile.

Sacramento City, California

April 22, 1850
My Dear Wife:

You ask when you may look for me home. I shall try merchandise, teaming, etc., in other words speculating, this summer, and perhaps next winter and then, ----I can tell you better. If I succeed in making a small pile and wish to make it larger, and like the country, when may I expect you here?

Mr. Fobes wishes to have his wife come here in the fall. How would you like to come with her? You could come by the Isthmus in October or November so as to have dry weather in the crossing to Panama.

East Cleveland, June 23, 1850

Dear Husband;

I believe that you promised when you left to return in 18 months. I hope you fulfill the promise. I will not say as some "California widows" that I would not come if you sent for me, that if you wanted me you might come after me (for I have not made up my mind about that yet) but I do say that I am anxious to have you return to Ohio before you locate anywhere.

May 18, 1851

My dear Huldah, you see that I write warmly but my words seem cold in comparison with my emotions --- emotions which are not of a transient, but of a permanent character and always the same whenever your image presents itself to my mind. Often I wonder why I left you and the question suggest itself whether any moderate amount of fortune which I can carry back with me, will counter-balance the absence for 2 or 3 years from your beloved society.

And sometimes odd thoughts come into my mind. Will she feel as well acquainted with me as formerly?

Until I hear from and until I see you, and I hope much longer, I shall remain, My dear Huldah, very Respectfully, very hopefully, very sincerely, and very Affectionately Yours.

S. Mathews

Reinnette finished reading the letters and sat quietly. When her mother returned, Reinnette asked her, "Did he return for her?"

"Yes," Mrs. Clark said, "He came back, eventually."

"Then... where was his failure mother?" Reinnette asked, "I don't understand."

Her mother had her hands on her hips, a familiar gesture when she was trying to make a point.

"He came back with only $10,000 dollars, Reinnette, and he risked his life for it. It was a fool's journey. Likely as not he could have been killed."

"But he came back," Reinnette said quietly, "He came back to her."

Mrs. Clark face flushed and seemed to increase in intensity until it was a bright red. Between clenched teeth she said, "Make no mistake, young lady, he came back but you don't have that option. If you leave, if you take off with this... this uneducated flight instructor, you're closing the door on this family. Permanently. You will not be accepted here again. It will be as if you never existed to us."

Reinnette's eyes flashed angrily, then she felt tears forming. She would not be held hostage to the wealth, or the position in life or the control that her family was trying to exert upon her. Grandfather Mathews had shown courage, at the very least. Her mother was the one that was afraid. All of them were in hiding. This mansion, this opulence, was nothing more than a castle that in keeping the world out, held them prisoners within.

"I'm leaving," Reinnette said.

"Fine." And her mother left the room.

Reinnette and Richard moved to California, and within a short time Reinnette had acquired her commercial pilot's license, just following Amelia Earheart. Eventually, they purchased a ranch near Chico and raised three children.

Reinnette never had contact with her family from the day she left, and when her parents died, the family fortune was, presumably, divided amongst the other children.

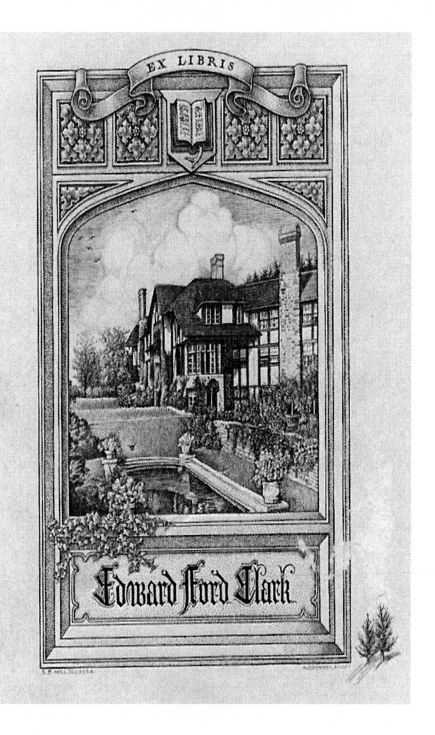

Chapter Fourteen

Let's go adventure then, just you and I
And stretch ourselves like eagles in an air
Too thin for wings of substance, in a sky
Of Stars and holes and empty places.
Shattered suns by wingtip traces,
Wheel and split antipodal.
Dip and soar on multimodal
Tentacles of mist;
Embrace and plummet,
Crease the vacuum, probe and search
And rise and camber into air.

A pair of travelers gliding back to where
There was nothing there before
But scattered empty shells.

"There was a time or two at the top of a mountain, or coursing down a river so remote that the last humans there built sod houses, or some times they fought it out with 600 lbs of animal in its own environment, or reviving a critter after a first time surgical procedure that I invented and then watching the moment of transformation, or sailing through a hurricane that lost all other craft at sea in the area or seeing the outcome of months of research and knowing for a moment, just for a single, silent moment, something that no one else on earth ever knew, or knows or will know until I tell them. The times when the most has been asked of you and you did it," Tom said in reflection. Rennie was listening and then Tom continued, "These are the things I think about in my life, the experiences I value most." Tom looked over to her, "What about you Rennie? What are the things that you reflect about? Value the most?"

Tom and Rennie were sailing in the Sea of Cortez on their sailboat, Shanti, which in Hindu means "the peace that passes all understanding." Shanti was a twenty-five foot Bristol Star. She had been selected and purchased since she had plenty of headroom and a large berth. The boat, combined with their Dodge Caravan that they converted to be self-contained, made for simple, yet comfortable living.

Shanti was the perfect boat to sleep on, especially during the warm seasons, so they took advantage of the weather by spending their nights just lying in the v-birth listening to the rhythmic sound of the halyards as they tapped against the mast.

This time of the year was warm, and the stars were so bright you could reach up and touch them, Rennie often thought. She had heard others say that before, but never really knew what it meant until they were there in the Sea of Cortez, just the two of them, getting up with the sunrise in order to not miss one precious minute of the next day.

They started their honeymoon by testing Shanti in the warm waters of the Bay of San Carlos, originally intending to sail for a couple of weeks and then return to the states to begin their sojourn around the entire country. After that, they assumed they would probably end up somewhere in the Caribbean. Both were free now from their professorships and retired. Their children were grown, and they were eager to begin their lives together. Lives that would be lived in marked contrast to the hardships of the past.

Rennie smiled back at Tom and turned her wine glass around in her hands in contemplation. Her brown hair hung down around her shoulders in two, long braids and framed her high cheekbones. With her lovely olive skin she could have passed for American Indian to most observers.

Her feet were propped up on the small seating area of the cockpit and Tom was sitting across from her smiling. He was holding the tiller and watching the sail. Shanti was more drifting than sailing in the small breeze that headed them across the San Carlos Bay in the Sea of Cortez. Tom began a slow starboard tack and said to Rennie, "Commin' about Rennie." He turned the tiller and the boom smoothly switched sides. The sail grew taut after Tom adjusted the mainsheet in Shanti's cleat, and the boat increased its speed through the warm water. Rennie's hand hung over the side as she tried to feel the spray from the wake.

She looked past Tom toward the shore. It was breathtakingly beautiful and she was once again overwhelmed with a sudden rush of love for this man. She became filled with an inner joy that she had never experienced before and she couldn't seem to stop smiling.

He was everything to her and had been since she first laid eyes on him.

Up until now, her life had been anything but easy, too many failed relationships, too many unreasonable expectations from her family to live up to. Now, she felt, it was her time at last.

Sitting on their sailboat, Rennie couldn't help but think back and remember herself as a child sailing her little dory off the shore at her family's summer home in Hyannis Port so many years ago. She had always been a good sailor. She had grown up spending summers on the New England coast, and of her many recreations, sailing had been a favorite. Her parents had given to her a small boat of her own when she was just a child. She taught herself to sail, and as she grew more confident, she could be found on her small boat continuously during the summer, even in the rougher weather off the New England coast. Storms didn't frighten her, and she was able to handle even the harshest conditions.

Tom was also a competent sailor, having learned during college on the Great Lakes of Michigan. Combined, they made for a crew that could handle nearly anything, which was fortunate, as their skills were frequently needed to survive the sudden storms that had a way of cropping up in the Sea of Cortez.

Rennie sometimes wondered about her life, it had all rushed by so quickly. She had begun to believe that she would drift through the rest of her years alone, and she had come to accept that. Yet now, life had taken an unexpected turn for the better. Rennie looked at Tom and she knew, deep within her heart, that she would spend the rest of her life with this man. It amused her that he didn't look like what she imagined the 'love of her life' would look like, *should* he ever come along. She was forever thrilled by the strange magic that makes you love and adore one person, yet not another.

Now, at the age of sixty, she found herself head over heels in love, able to experience feelings of adoration that she never dreamed were still possible, the 'walking into walls' kind of love. Once, she caught herself staring into space not too long after she met Tom, just staring for no reason at all and with a smile on her face. She was sitting in the college cafeteria near some other professors in between classes when it happened. But what she knew that the other professors, who smiled as they passed and raised their eyebrows at her, could not know, was that all the space she was staring into was filled with Tom, every bit of it, and she could almost reach out into that space and touch his face, hold him close and melt his body into her own.

How and why she was so fortunate to find someone and be able to fall so completely in love at her age, she could not fathom. All she knew or needed to know was that the touch of his hand on hers was enough to make her weak in the knees. That was enough for her, she thought…that was certainly enough for a sixty-year-old lady.

Her mind returned to the conversation and she tried to answer Tom's question about what her favorite things might be, her own "mountaintop experiences" in life. She knew what he meant, had heard him speak of his own favorite things and admired them, but hers were not the same.

There was no doubt in her mind, her favorite thing was him. All of him, everything about him from his exceptional, brilliant mind to just the way he looked at her. Oh, she thought, she had a few wonderful experiences during her life, her commercial pilots' license for one, summers at their cottage in Hyannis Port that now belonged to the Kennedy family, but they paled in comparison to the goose bumps she felt as she looked into his blue eyes or listened to him speak. Even the way he walked was perfect to her. Her heart soared with the knowledge that he loved her the same way. This very capable, loving, bright man loved her just as she did him. Finally, life was too good to be true. Maybe these feelings were available to her because she was a woman, but no, not at this stage of her life. She knew Tom loved her just as deeply. In her moments of doubt, she said to herself, "Rennie, just accept where you are, your good fortune and enjoy it. No need to try to figure out why, just relax and enjoy."

She took a sip of her wine and said, "Tom, I'd love to be philosophical and tell you some marvelous, splendid thing or things that have happened, but to tell you the truth, the very best thing that has ever happened to me in my life has been you. Oh, I know, that probably sounds trite, but at the risk of boring you to death, I'm afraid it's true." She smiled and her voice caught in her throat as she tried to continue, "You are the love of my life. I never dreamed I'd be lucky enough to find someone like you to love, and that's the simple truth." Overcome with emotion, Rennie wiped the tears from her brown eyes with her long fingertips.

They watched the sunset that night wrapped in each other's arms, gazing in wonder together with mist filled eyes as the sun dipped into the ocean over the Baja peninsula. It was to be only one of an indeterminate number of sunsets they would enjoy together over the next several years.

Originally they had thought they would be testing Shanti out for a couple of weeks and then moving on, but the more they sailed around the beautiful waters of the Bay of San Carlos, the more Tom and Rennie found Mexico fascinating.

There was a perfect harbor, complete with a tiny marina and a trailer park with a restaurant, and they had befriended the owners. As they sailed and bumped all around the gorgeous bay, picnicking on the beautiful white sand beaches and exalting in the glory of the warm water, they fell more and more in love with Mexico and decided to stay instead of leaving for the Caribbean.

So, it was, their lives together had begun. It was a new journey, a time of discovery in all aspects for the both of them. They discovered new areas to explore, new places to see and most of all, they continually rediscovered their love for each other.

After a time, they came to realize that San Carlos, apart from all of Mexico, was hard to leave. They still intended to explore, so they decided it could serve as a base to which they could return. After some investigation and some humorous, yet sobering stories about the complications of building a house in Mexico, they decided to take the challenge. Both Tom and Rennie became fluent in Spanish. They realized it would be foolish to attempt a project of this nature unless they could barter and argue in the native tongue. And it was fun. Attending a course at the Language Institute gave them some intellectual stimulation. Since they had both spent a lifetime learning, they welcomed the chance to remain sharp.

As they searched for the ideal location, they chanced upon a place just south of San Carlos, called "Area Rustica." It was close enough to the town to provide convenient shopping, yet there was privacy and seclusion. Further searches yielded some competent help and soon they were excavating and laying a foundation. The house itself had several unique features, one of which was the master bedroom. Remaining cool in the heat of summer was always a challenge in Mexico and air conditioning was difficult to come by, so the bedroom was actually a tunnel built into a rocky Cliffside. The rest of the house was made of adobe, which was known to keep a place cool in the hotter days, yet provided adequate insulation in the winter.

The project started on a small scale yet continued to grow as Tom and Rennie let their imaginations run wild. Eventually, they ended up with a Spanish Villa, complete with a courtyard in the center and a fireplace next to the spacious dining and kitchen area. It took time to build, but time was one thing they had.

For the sake of sanity, they made sure they took frequent breaks, sometimes leaving for weeks to explore and sail, but always they found themselves anxious to return and pick up where they had left off. When it was finally finished, Rennie planted an elaborate garden in the courtyard and grew vegetables. It amazed her that in such a tropical climate, where everything would grow so well, there were few fresh vegetables for sale in the local markets. In time she had such abundance that she made a habit of taking bushels of ripe tomatoes into the poorer areas and giving them away. It gained her considerable favor in the community, although she never really thought about it selfishly. There was more than they needed, it simply made sense to her to give.

The local Mexicans found both Tom and Rennie fascinating. Unabashed about their lives, Tom and Rennie lived as they pleased. Rennie, in fact, had a habit of gardening in the nude until Tom noticed that there were several young boys who would sneak peeks through the holes in the fences. He repaired the holes and attempted to convince Rennie that she was, just possibly, being a distraction, but she cared little about it. She was a free spirit and believed in living as you choose and Tom could find little fault in that. In fact it was one of the things he admired most about her.

When the Villa was completely finished and they were satisfied, it was time to begin some serious exploration. They prepared the van and purchased a portable boat that folded into a snug package, which they strapped to the outside.

They decided to attempt to circumnavigate Central America and explore the remote, uncharted areas. They left and traveled hundreds of miles, stopping when something attracted their interest, and then staying until they were ready to go on.

At the border of Belize they were turned back. Their vehicle description didn't match the van they were driving since they had changed since entering Mexico, so they were denied access.

It didn't concern them, however. They just turned North up the eastern coast of Mexico and continued, bumping along old highways and poking into every corner. On their stops, they camped and fished and most of all, relaxed. When they became restless, they explored, and on several occasions happened upon pyramids, many of which were not on the maps. Tom became engrossed with pyramids. He would take Rennie up the steps, often through tangled vines that had to be cleared away each step. These were ancient ruins and Tom and Rennie tried to decipher the hieroglyphics they found etched in stone stairways. Combining their intellects, they made progress on occasion, and Rennie watched bemused as Tom paced around the symbols, muttering to himself about the significance of the serpent to aboriginal tribes. Later, when they traveled near the coast, they assembled their portable boat and explored remote beaches.

One evening they were startled, as their campsite was visited unexpectedly. They were camped on a white sand beach that was backed by very heavy jungle. They had paddled their little boat around a point when they found the spot, far too enticing to pass up, so they beached and went ashore and made camp.

The sounds of tropical birds rang out in the late afternoon and they had just settled down to cook dinner and watch the sun set behind the mountains in the west. There wasn't a civilized area for miles, and as they prepared the meal, they looked up just in time to see a scantily clad man walking out of the jungle. He carried a primitive bow and walked toward them without taking any notice of their presence. He moved calmly to within ten feet of where they were sitting, not altering his course, and then on down to the water where he crouched on his knees and became totally motionless. Suddenly, he raised his bow, and drew it to his shoulder and shot an arrow. He got up slowly, walked over to the edge of the jungle and after rustling around in the bushes for a moment, he returned walking by them carrying a small deer over his shoulders.

He never looked at them, he just continued back towards the part of the jungle from where he had first appeared, and then he was gone. Tom and Rennie felt as though they had witnessed an incident from the ancient past. It was as if they were time-travelers and had been given a vision in some mystical way.

They traveled further north and later finally camped back on the western coast of Mexico just north of San Blas. They loved it there and became involved and friendly with some of the permanent residents, in particular, with a couple that was known for their generosity to the residents who were in need.

Fishing was so good in those days, especially off shore and out by the islands, that there was always more than enough to share. Tom and Rennie could not store much, so they gave generously.

Before long they became acquainted with several of the locals and were secretly told that a very important day was fast approaching. A small band of Indians that lived some distance away in the mountains would be coming down to bathe in the ocean for their yearly religious ceremony. The ceremony itself evolved around the moon at a certain phase that coincided with other omens within the tribe. It seemed that this particular band was thought to be remnants of the Indians that were forced off the islands many years before. They had been dumped on shore where they had retreated into the mountains in fear for their lives. Now, the few of them that were left lived far away from any sort of civilization and only came into town once a year, primarily for their religious ceremony and to trade for a few supplies.

Tom and Rennie were absolutely fascinated and when they were asked if they would like to meet them, they enthusiastically agreed. They were told they could not take pictures, as the Indians believed the flash would steal their souls, thus rendering any further spiritual trips to the ocean pointless. The only thing they would be allowed to do was to give the adults' coins and nothing else. Not even food would be accepted, and certainly, nothing was to be given to the children, as they didn't want them to even *know* the concept of begging.

Finally, the day came when the natives were supposed to appear out of the jungle that surrounds San Blas, yet none arrived. It was terribly disappointing. Then another day and another went by and everyone began to think something awful had happened to the little tribe. Then one morning they came. They were dressed in their finest garb, and they looked almost as colorful as the women of Guatemala who dress in their brightest attire when they marched down the trails of the mountains with baskets of coffee on their heads. Bright reds and yellows with bands of blue, all set against the lush green of the mountain jungles behind them.

The Indians came as a small band down the jungle trails out of the mountains in the same manner and in the same colors, but without the coffee, and Tom and Rennie were amazed at how bright and polished they looked.

They were physically beautiful people and the children were as scrubbed and clean as any alter boy on Palm Sunday. Olive skinned and bright, white teeth with smiles from ear to ear; the tribe was obviously delighted to see everyone again.

Some of the town residents must have been old friends as they greeted each other as though they were long lost relatives. There were about twenty-two of them altogether, with about eight or nine children ranging from the ages of three to early teens, and none of them were over five feet tall. They looked completely different than any race Tom and Rennie had ever seen. Not American Indian, Mexican or even Hawaiian, but they had their own unique look, and they carried themselves with a friendly openness that told of a beautiful culture.

The Indians visited with friends and tried to speak to everyone, but their language was completely different than the Spanish spoken in that area, so communication was largely limited to sign language. It was obvious that this tribe had been completely isolated from the rest of the world.

As they were introduced to Tom and Rennie, they very politely smiled and offered their hands in the symbolic Western gesture, a gesture they had learned of, but one that was completely meaningless to them. After a few moments they began to move away toward the center of town, and as quickly as they came into view, they were gone.

Toms' friends told him the natives would be in San Blas for a little while and then at sunset they would go to a special place at the shore's edge where they would take their clothes off and perform their religious ceremony. It would take about an hour, and after that, they would disappear back into the jungle on their way to their home.

Tom asked where they lived, where their camp was and if they migrated, but the answer was that no one knew and even if they did, they wouldn't tell for fear of invasion of the tribe's privacy. Seclusion was all this little band of displaced Indians had left, and the town of San Blas protected them as best they could and simply looked forward to their yearly visits.

After leaving the area surrounding San Blas and bidding farewell to their friends, Tom and Rennie set out again in search of other sights. Rennie loved nothing more than soaking in a hot spring of any kind, and so many of their sojourns were spent tracing down the "agua caliente" or any reasonable facsimile. On one trip while on the western side of lower Mexico they gleefully followed a lead given to them by the owner of a tiny market in one of the small towns. He had seen signs years ago along a deserted road that was supposed to lead to an ancient hot spring. Rennie went into 'full point' and Tom laughed and agreed to the adventure. They drove for miles and the road became more and more narrow and then finally stopped altogether. Eventually, they came face to face with a jungle so thick you would need ten machetes to go three feet. Rennie was truly disappointed, and when they stopped at the next town, the owner of another small store said, "No, senor, there hasn't been water of any kind there for over 1000 years."

Yet as they continued on during this same exploration, they came upon enormous rock heads carved into shapes of a nationality of men Tom had never seen before. The rocks were almost completely covered in vines and growth. Tom and Rennie were surprised that they even spotted them. They took the time to pull the vines off to get a better look, and the only conclusion they could come to was that they were of Mayan origin. It was not a hot spring, yet it seemed well worth the journey regardless.

Tom was once again fascinated by the stone heads and discussed the discovery with Rennie at length. She was interested as well, but not to the same degree, which surprised Tom. He felt, however, that the loss of soaking in some nice, hot water in the wilderness was too great a loss in Rennie's mind.

Not long after this final discovery, the sojourn drew to a close. They had been away from their home in San Carlos for several months and were anxious to be in familiar surroundings again. On the way back, they briefly visited the Museum of Anthropology in Mexico City and Tom spoke with the curator there. Tom felt it his obligation to share some of the discoveries, and the museum became extremely interested. Some of the discoveries were original, and Tom's depth of understanding impressed them. Rennie participated, but soon became disinterested in archaeology. It surprised Tom, as she had usually been the driving force in the journey. However, he reasoned, she was getting tired and it was time to rest. They started back and after three days pulled into San Carlos and collapsed, exhausted, in their home.

Several years passed, and Tom and Rennie kept themselves busy working on the Villa and taking small trips. There were few places in Mexico by now that they had not seen, but they still liked to get away, if for no other reason than to break the routine. They sometimes sailed for a few days in the Sea of Cortez, and on alternate trips they would drive the van into the hills or deserts, making sure they had seen it all. They were happy and time passed quickly.

Tom was always ready to go. He relished the idea of getting back into travel and away from the daily chores that seemed to grow monotonous, but Rennie became more and more resistant. Tom wondered about this, as she would make excuses for staying home, sometimes stating that the garden needed tending and her precious plants would suffer in her absence. Yet when they did stay home, she spent little time in the garden. She might be found in it, but instead of caring for the wilting tomatoes, she would sit near them and pick at the buds, pinching them off and casting them listlessly on the ground. Tom felt a burgeoning concern, but reconciled himself to the fact that she was ten years older than he and deserved to rest and relax. Tom let her be and spent his time keeping occupied with the boat and the maintenance of the house. Yet something kept nagging him in his mind. It was a persistent thought, and one that he tried to shut out. Rennie seemed different in some way. She didn't seem the same, not herself, and try as he might, he couldn't explain it.

Sometimes she was listless and unfocused, and when they sailed their boat, she, the consummate sailor, would often forget to tie lines off or to properly trim the sails.

Tom watched and rationalized. He could easily pass it off as a form of eccentricity, God knew they both had their fair share of that, but this seemed qualitatively different.

He was ready, at one point, to ask her if there was a problem with their relationship. It was an idea that he could not possibly even imagine, yet his morbid curiosity got the best of him.

Before he had the chance to ask, Rennie spoke up one day out of the clear blue sky. "Tom, I want to go home," she said.

"Home?" Tom said, "But this *is* our home, here, in San Carlos."

"No," Rennie said, "I want to go back home to California." Tom could tell she was disturbed and absolutely serious, so after a brief pause, he relented.

"Alright," he said, "We'll sell the house and go back."

Within the year they had sold the villa and their beloved Shanti and moved back to California. They settled into a small cottage in the town of Los Osos, which was only a few miles from Morro Bay where Tom had spent time on a houseboat years before. Rennie seemed satisfied and Tom was happy about it. They had said their goodbyes to their dear friends in Mexico and it was painful, but to see Rennie happy once again more than compensated.

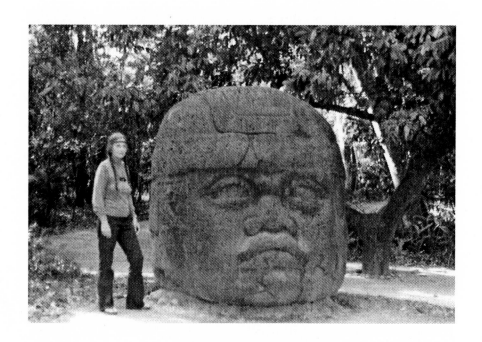

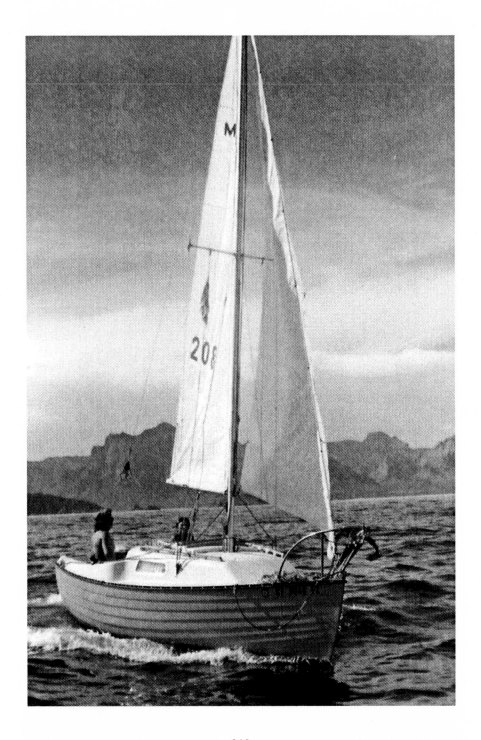

Chapter Fifteen

...and she lurches across the threshold.
eyes wide and wild as a startled coon.
One hand clings to a clutch of leaves,
ragged souvenirs of autumn.
"Night," she screams, hurling leaves in the air.
Oh God Night Again!"
She begins to tremble
bits of leaves drifting to the floor.
She kneels, strokes the carpet
grabbing the fragments.

Tom and Rennie returned to Los Osos and settled back into their home. Fortunately, they had kept their little cottage while they lived in Mexico for eleven years and now it came in handy.

Tom carried a growing burden of concern for Rennie, yet early on he lived in denial over the serious nature of her condition. Even during the ensuing worst times as her disease progressed, his love for Rennie and for their privacy kept him from asking for help until he had no choice.

He held much of what happened during those beginning years inside, preferring to feel, not think, that her actions existed only in some Valhalla of nascent state. Their lives remained private for the most part, yet ultimately he revealed everything in its entirety to a few friends, but not until it was over. Until then, only his closest friends and family knew what Tom and Rennie had gone through.

It could be surmised, with a certain amount of reliability, that when Tom finally faced the inevitable conclusion that Rennie had Alzheimer's, he would in retrospect have taken an entirely different path, one that was far better traveled in those days.

But the easy well-traveled path had never been his way, and after he caught his breath and accepted the facts as they were, he prepared to engage in battle once again in his life. This time the life he would be fighting for was not his own. This time it would be for someone he loved with every fiber of his being, and this battle would prove to be his most challenging. He would have to call upon his vast background in research, and somehow find a way to save her. It would require dedication, love and faith, something that in combination, he hoped, could perhaps work a miracle.

A miracle, in fact, was what was needed.

Dr. Law tells his recollection of the ordeal....

"It was after we had returned from our eleven years in Mexico to Los Osos. We were getting up there in years, especially Rennie, as she is about ten years older than I am, and we had just about run out of intellectual things to do there. We had seen it all.

Not long after we were home, a good friend of mine lost his wife to Alzheimer's. She had been diagnosed at a fairly early age and only lasted about ten years. My friend, for some odd reason I thought, kept telling me that he felt Rennie had early signs of Alzheimer's. I can't tell you how much I resented his saying that. She did not. She was just a little forgetful, as we all are from time to time as we advance in age. I should know, shouldn't I? Me, the absent minded professor. Still, my friend persisted over time and I was just as adamant in the other direction. There wasn't anything wrong except...except that eventually, as her actions became even more 'odd' to my way of thinking, I was forced to assume something really *was* wrong.

Finally, my friend insisted I go with him to an Alzheimer's support group meeting. I attended several times and listened carefully. There was no resemblance, I thought, between the behaviors and problems these caregivers described and the frankly psychotic behavior of my wife. I refused to describe my problems in the group because Rennie wasn't Alzheimer's and I... I didn't have any problems...

Backing up, our story begins twenty-six years ago. Rennie was 60, and I was 50 then. She had one more year to go until retirement, so for that year I became a househusband. It was a romantic year, one in which we could focus on each other. We lived in a home on the cliff's edge at Pismo Beach. The entire western wall of the house was glass. Rennie's office was in her bed, so on weekends she would lie there grading papers and preparing classes on the edge of the world.

It was a perfect time in our lives to meet. Our careers and all their busyness and preoccupations were behind us. Our children were all grown, and we were healthy and young enough to still be bold, full of adventure, experimental and vital. We met in a class I was teaching, partly as a joke, in the Open University in San Luis Obispo. It was a massage class and there is a story and a smile in that, but there isn't time here. Despite serious effort on both our parts not to, we fell in love right away, and it deepened over the subsequent years.

We married. We honeymooned for two weeks in a 24-foot sailboat in the San Juan Islands. Rennie got her motorcycle license. We honeymooned again on a motorcycle tour of the Gold Country. She retired. We bought an eighteen-foot trailer sailboat and set off to circumnavigate the United States, launching, 'Shanti' everywhere we felt like it, but aiming to a Florida launch and a cruise to the Bahamas. I was an experienced deep-sea sailor and navigator, Rennie was a skilled sailor. Rennie mostly knew navigation from her flying experience. She picked up sea piloting in one session, in about a half an hour or so. We loaded up and set off on our tour. But first, because it was close and underpopulated and good sea cruising, why not test the boat in the sea of Cortez? So we drove to Mexico, launched the boat and stayed for eleven years.

In those eleven years we lived a lifetime of adventure. We circled the whole country of Mexico in a van, staying on beaches and in villages with the residents, visiting Shamans, matriculating at the language institute, making friends with Mayan young people. We cruised the Caribbean coast in a six-foot folding dinghy, locating and exploring nearly every ruin in Mexico, even the notorious Palenque with the magic mushrooms, one of which we found exploring while on a Honda trail motorcycle we used, but we had to come back another time to be able to remember the place.

The point I hope to make in this narrative is to portray a vibrant mature woman, full of life, curiosity, courage and vitality, fearless and insatiable for living and for new experiences. And, I think now that I can look back on it, that may have been where it began. In Mexico we had built a large home on an acre of land by the Sea of Cortez. One day she said, 'I am through going to sea.' I was dismayed and shocked. We had just bought a new sailboat, a perfect heavy-weather cruising boat, ideal for our risk taking voyages, and we had a great native ponga with a 40 hp outboard that we took big game fishing 25-30 miles out to sea. It was a mystery, wholly out of character, wholly discordant with all our plans, our life style. Her reason was, 'I am too old and I am tired of pulling up anchors.'

Within a year we had folded everything and moved back to Los Osos, to a one-bedroom cottage, no ranch, no garden, no boats and no friends. Maybe it began then. Maybe I should have known. But I didn't. Not then, not later, not through the most tempestuous transformations of character. I could not believe what was not possible.

There were probably signs much earlier than that. Not many years after we were married, Rennie became deeply involved with a religious cult, which was part Hindu, part Christian, part New Age and which managed to completely miss the point of all three. It was specious. It was superficial. It was banal. It was fatuous, in the worst tradition of Edgar A. Guest. And, above all, it was enormously financially successful. Rennie went to retreats two or three times a year, which sounded drearily ascetic. Long hours of meditation, days of vows of silence, vegetarian food, no alcohol and no sex. Dreary. But she entered into it a long way, becoming some equivalent of a priestess, going on pilgrimages to India, Israel and Italy.

She maintained this involvement after we moved back to Los Osos, some thirteen years ago. It was discordant with her unremarkable Episcopalian background, but then so was she. At the onset of what we shall call, 'The Crisis,' she lost all interest and has never brought it up since. Recently, I asked her what it was all about; she replied, 'I was looking for help.'

Then there was a period about nine or ten years ago when she became very distressed at the content of movies. Suspense or horror films scared her into spasms. It was necessary to screen content before exposing her to them, and even then, we sometimes had to leave the movie somewhere in the middle.

At that time I was writing quite a lot, fiction, poetry, essays, philosophy. I even wrote a book titled *Modern Poetry for People Who Hate Poetry*.

Rennie was supportive, for a while. Then suddenly she became extremely distressed at some views I had written on religious issues. She complained to a mutual friend that she 'had no idea I thought that way,' whereas in fact, she was well acquainted with my views on that and all other subjects, and the friend told her so. He knew as she did, that I had openly held these views from long before we met and throughout our marriage. She became so terribly, disproportionately disturbed that I stopped writing altogether and only resumed a few years ago.

Perhaps that was a sign and I should have caught it. But I didn't even suspect. At about that time Rennie took an evening course at Cuesta College on potted plant cultivation. She had always been an avid and prolifically successful gardener. She devoted a lot of time and concentration to it. Our lot was too small in Los Osos and too crowded with tree roots from neighboring land to raise anything in the soil. The potted plants were the answer to the problem. She began collecting and raising plants....lots of plants in lots of pots. She never saw a plant she didn't love. They were all orphans and she was in the wholesale adopting mode. At the time of the crisis, my son cleaned out most, but by no means all, of the plants in the house. Remember, this is a one-bedroom house, 890 sq. feet in all. There are larger trailers. His count of potted plants removed from the living room alone was 160. In all, from the whole tiny house, he extracted 350 potted plants.

Was this a sign? Was it obsessive compulsive behavior, beyond ordinary eccentricity in the elderly? Although I did feel it was somewhat excessive enthusiasm for a hobby, I didn't think of it as pathological. For one thing, I was deeply grateful she wasn't into puppies.

There is no doubt there were other signs and symptoms, other bellwethers along the way. Like the foregoing, maybe I should have caught onto them, but I ignored them. Rennie is an extraordinary person and it is easy to dismiss the extraordinary in such a person until the extraordinary imperceptibly merges into the bizarre. And so it became.

I think in retrospect it began about eight or nine years ago when Rennie fell ill with a mysterious malady. She escalated a fever; her liver enzymes rocketed out of the normal range. We were referred to a hematologist. By the time we got to his office, Rennie was in atrial fibrillation. She spent eleven days in the hospital while a parade of specialists, even a tropical disease specialist, ran a battery of tests. She was visibly and dangerously ill almost the entire time.

No diagnosis was ever achieved. The consensus was that her immune system had failed, but no one knew why. The evidence was so strong though that we were both tested for AIDS. They were preparing to do a liver biopsy when, just as mysteriously as she fell ill, she began to recover. We went home, I nursed her for a couple of months and she was apparently well.

But now, again in retrospect, I surmise that the Alzheimer's dates from this illness. I don't know. I only suspect. If it was a result of some systemic infection, she easily could have brought it back with her from her trip to India, Israel or Italy. Who could know?

Sometimes, in our darkest nights, we look deep into ourselves to attempt to establish and determine when a certain significant event first occurred. It is a natural process for all of us as human beings and remains a vain attempt to reverse what already is in effect and traceable to a definite cause. We ask ourselves if we could have changed anything by the knowing…the answer is, obviously, and quite frankly, no. Certainly some things are preordained and are not changeable in the path of life, nor, perhaps, should they be.

As students of the origin and development of mind/brain we quite properly devote significant energy to the study of the development of mental expression in infancy and childhood. It seems to me that there is much to be learned too as that process reverses itself, as the 'modules' of brain function decline and dwindle with the erosion of aging. Toward that end I tried to find landmarks in the loss of mental integrity in the only population presently available to me, my wife.

Now, sometimes there are pensive moments when I try to think back to where, in the evolution of Rennie's dementia, some hint of what was to come may first have peeked through. Mostly these reflections are overstuffed with moments and incidents of 'maybe, but maybe not' sorts of recollections. But recently a memory has emerged of an incident that menaced our relationship some, and appeared soon after we returned to this country, around the summer of 1986. At the time, the incident appeared to point up a profound difference in our outlooks on life.

There is a species of butterfly, a lovely orange and black migrant, popularly known as the Gulf Fritillary. This tiny traveler crosses the Gulf of Mexico annually to seek out growths of the passion vine, a fairly common, although not abundant, native species in the Southwest. The Fritillary needs the passion vine to lay its eggs on. Its larvae can feed on no other plant. Unquestionably there is a symbiotic relationship that benefits the plant as well, though I don't recall the details at the moment. Because of the ease and reliability of this relationship, it serves with some charm as an illustration of plant/animal interrelations.

To introduce Rennie to this natural pageant, I bought a passion vine and planted it just outside the dining area window where the little drama was framed on the stage three feet beyond us with every meal. Eventually, not long after the leaves appeared really, the butterflies arrived early, and in numbers that surprised even me, one who had some previous experience with these Lepidopterons.

Eggs were deposited predictably, and in the natural order of things, the larvae emerged. They brought a color and pattern of their own, pretty in its own way, but bearing no recognizable relationship to the parent's ornamentation. As they contentedly munched their way across the foliage, a conflict began to appear. Whatever had hatched, and in contrast with the leaves, was identifiable, Rennie at some time or another went outdoors and one by one pinched each caterpillar to death.

I was aghast at this. She explained she didn't like the worms destroying her plant. I went over again that the reason for buying the plant was to attract the butterflies, and it was absurd to do that without encouraging them to consummate the reproductive cycle that drew them to the host plant in the first place.

Over and over, she went out, often at night, and killed the larvae. Over and over I explained the symbiosis, the reason for having the plant. Reason never prevailed. The slaughter and the protestation cum explanation persisted in tandem for several weeks until one day, while I was away, Rennie took the pruning saw and hacked the passion vine off at ground level.

She couldn't see the butterfly for the worm...I should have known then.

Just after the last illness, about eight years ago, when Rennie came home to recuperate, our oldest friend and the person who married us said of Rennie, 'something is missing.'

One year later, almost exactly, Rennie again fell seriously ill and was hospitalized. Again, no one could find the cause. Again she was discharged after a couple of weeks and again with no diagnosis. Once more her immune system seemed to have failed her. But while in the hospital, serious pneumonitis took hold and nearly finished her. This time it took longer to nurse her back to health and activity, but she made it.

I feel to this day that whatever compromised her immune system to the harm of her liver once, and her lungs the second time, continued on to her brain. I realize that this is equivalent to an infectious theory of the etiology of Alzheimer's, and that is not the presently favored explanation. I realize also that it's a one-shot guess, but good research is often born of less.

Rennie had been worried for some time about her memory. We spoke to our physician about it. He asked the old chestnut questions, like 'who is the president of the United States? What day is it?' She answered them all correctly and he dismissed her concern.

Now I think I should have taken her more seriously. She was closer to the problem than he.

Following her hospitalization with immune failure, Rennie became even more concerned about her memory or its loss. She complained about it to the hepatologist, who acknowledged her concern and ordered an NMRI. I saw the film from that myself and agreed with the radiologist there was no sign of the cortical white spots typical of Alzheimer's. There was shrinkage, but we lose brain cells at the rate of thousands per day; in eighty years, one shouldn't be surprised that the volume of the brain has been reduced by the massive emigration.

Rennie's concern persisted. We were referred to a costly series of ineffective treatments. We went to psychologists, to memory therapists, women's groups, age groups....everybody, even to a sort of gerontologist, whose blood tests were negative, as was yet another NMRI.

Memory loss is a signal flag in Alzheimer's. We were right to suspect it. But of the ten signs of Alzheimer's, two were all she ever displayed, one of them being moderate memory loss, the other being problems with numbers.

It's difficult to tell exactly when the depression began. But about nine years ago, while we were working on taxes, something catastrophic happened that gave it away. Rennie had always handled all our bookkeeping, all the investments and all the taxes. I hated that sort of thing, wasn't good at it. She enjoyed it, felt it was part of her birthright and did it well. Why should I do badly something she did well? So, I confined my aid to creative cheating on taxes, back when it could be done.

Then one February, Rennie began an agitated pacing from our office in the garage to her files in the bedroom, carrying file folders. She became increasingly, exponentially agitated. When I asked what was wrong, she said she couldn't find some tax file. In fact, she couldn't find any of them. Suddenly we were two weeks from the tax interview and she had no records.

Nor could she manage to enter the right numbers in the right places, nor anything else to do with finances. Not even balance her checkbook. And BOOM, there I was, totally ignorant, inexperienced, untalented and completely bereft of any records to work from. Years later I found tax documents filed under 'vitamins.' You get the picture.

Now the depression moved in with a roar! Depression preempted the whole landscape of her mind. It saturated every moment of the day, like living downwind of a burning dump. Rennie was becoming increasingly aware of the tragedy that was pursuing her. Each time I would begin work on anything numerical - checkbook, taxes or investments - she would detonate hyperbolically. She would become extremely agitated, would rush back and forth through our tiny house, yelling, shrieking, ranting, pausing in the rush to berate me, then racing on, protesting, proclaiming and denouncing. Then, once in a while she would pause, ask to talk calmly with me a moment, and then when we were seated and focused, say something like, 'When did you stop loving me?'

These outbursts varied in frequency, though not much in intensity. They would happen three to four times a week when things were calm, but they would last up to 48 hours when they hit. Whenever there was 'provocation,' which is to say I was working on any of our affairs involving numbers, then these eruptions would happen as often as every day and last until peaking again the next day. One memorable day there was fully five totally hysterical eruptions, totally out of control, all directed at me.

Sometimes I would go out for a walk around the block. I was afraid to leave her longer than that. More often than not she would then pursue me down the street, sometimes not fully dressed, and howling the entire time. This went on without interruption for months - no, as I think about it, for years! It first happened when I suddenly had to take charge of the tax preparation. I subsequently spent part of December, all of January and February, for five years preparing tax records and every one of those years, throughout all those weeks, the hysterical agitation continued. And throughout it all, punctuating the uproar, was the endlessly relentless repetitive threat of suicide: 'I'm going to kill myself!'

It never let up.

Why didn't I see it then? I have a letter from the psychiatrist who was admitting and treating her at French hospital that said she was quite normal and in possession of all her faculties. Two days after that was signed, he readmitted her for the third time after a failed suicide attempt. I was being assured by the best medical advice I could get, Internists, Gerontologists, Psychiatrists all said that she was perfectly normal, just growing old and that she didn't have Alzheimer's.

Yet Rennie's weren't idle suicide threats. Several times she ran to her car and drove off shrieking that she was going to drive off a cliff on Highway 1. Many times she grabbed one of my kitchen knives and threatened to stab herself. After one instance when she nearly did, I installed locks on the knife drawers. That infuriated her and led to amplified and strident pledges to kill herself.

To add to the suicidal obsession, Rennie would frequently forget she was not to interfere with documents and would take whole handfuls of files out of my filing cabinets and refile them elsewhere. Eventually I had to install locks on all the filing cabinets, and you can imagine what that provoked. A real uproar ensued.

The mail was always a problem, and one way or another she managed to get it, and then whatever it was became lost forever.

Rennie knew, of course, what was happening to her mind. She could sense it; even index it in the slipping away of her competence in bookkeeping and accounting. She had been aware that her mind was ebbing for a long time, but now it was terrifying.

Throughout all these years we tried one resource after another to get Rennie some help. Now, with very real threats to kill her self, we had no choice. Psychiatric treatment was mandated by hospitalization for repeated suicide attempt and threat. Now, simultaneously, she was seeing Psychologists, counselors, therapists, support groups and Psychiatrists.

Antidepressant medication was prescribed at the outset, of course. Despite trying a whole pharmacopoeia of them, none ever did the slightest bit of good.

I still didn't see Alzheimer's, dementia or anything but depression; after all, she was tumultuously depressed, in spades. There was no doubt of that, and the physicians and psychologists continued to treat depression as the crucial and *only* disorder...after all, this was a time of hope. Depression could be cured...couldn't it?

Finally, her infatuation with suicide became open and public. I had to take her to the approved Psychiatrist, who said immediately that if she planned to kill herself when she left his office, he was legally obligated to commit her to the French hospital's neuropsychiatries unit. When he asked her directly if she planned to do it, she answered straightforwardly, 'YES.'

So, Rennie was committed to French NPI the first of many times. She was kept a week and sent home. Nothing was changed. Almost immediately the same behavior surfaced. Again she was hospitalized and again sent home in a week. On the third hospitalization they started her on an antidepressant, a SSRI on Friday, and sent her home Saturday. The uproar resumed immediately. Eighteen hours after she was discharged, I could take no more and went to the store two blocks away to get some milk and bread and camp out overnight somewhere. But I couldn't do it; I couldn't just leave her in tears and anguish, alternately pleading and harassing, so I went back home...gingerly. She was still standing in the driveway where I had left her

20 minutes before, but now blood was pouring from her fingers. She had slashed her wrists.

Back to French NPI, of course, but now there were problems. By their own admission they should not have discharged Rennie eighteen hours after a suicide attempt for which their only treatment was a medication that requires three to six weeks to take effect. Now there was serious talk of committing her to a locked facility under extreme restraints. One could see that the professional personnel had turned completely around backwards in a synchronized effort to cover their own asses.

To me, the commitment had some appeal…but not nearly enough. However my beleaguered state might be calling out for relief, her anguish beggared my pain and I could not abandon her. So I got her released one more time.

Throughout all of this I had no idea that Alzheimer's was involved. And to compound the denial, I had no awareness of the effect this horror was having on me. A friend, with more insight and more experience than I, took me to an Alzheimer's support group. I attended several times and listened carefully. There was no resemblance, I thought, between the behaviors and problems these caregivers described and the frankly psychotic behavior of my wife. I refused to describe my problems in the group because Rennie wasn't Alzheimer's and I … I didn't have any problems. Then one week when the holocaust at home had escalated for 48 hours without interruption, I spoke…and it all rolled out. I have no idea what I said, but it was a torrent unleashed. The session was hushed and broke up right afterwards.

Four days later, when Rennie had perfected her trick of waking me seconds after I fell asleep for another tirade, after this had gone on for three days and nights with no rest, no sleep, no meals, no end - I tried to kill myself.

I had saved, as a last resort, the number of the suicide prevention hotline. Rennie had been relentlessly harping on the suicide tune for three days and nights at the least. I remember dialing the hotline, listening to a sleepy voice answer, and suddenly saying to Rennie, 'Dammit, stop all this pointless threatening; let me SHOW you how to do it right.' I took from its hiding place a 50-caliber revolver, loaded one chamber, spun the cylinder, placed the muzzle in my mouth and pulled the trigger. Click. I think that made me angry. I loaded another chamber, spun the cylinder again, pointed it at my uvula and pulled again. Click again. I loaded again, pulled again. Click again. Altogether I had loaded and fired 4 times without ever hitting a live round.

At that time, the police drove up and it was all over.... in a different way than it would have been one minute later.

That pretty much put an end to temporizing. I was, for the most part, out of the game. Clearly, professional care had to be found for Rennie and the locked facility was not an option. I would not sign for it, then or ever - and this is when things began to turn around.

Rennie's youngest son drove over from the valley and picked her up. For the next week his life was a shocked uproar, but he kept her a week. This gave me time to call Emily Hardford and find a care facility, FCF, that could handle someone as catastrophically affected as Rennie. Emile suggested Farrell Crest in Arroyo Grande. I liked the location because Rennie could not walk out and go home afoot, as she might have were she any closer. Of the owners of Farrell Crest, the husband was an RN and the wife was a counselor with seven years experience with addicts in withdrawal. But would they accept Rennie? Their facility was nearly full of typical Alzheimer's patients, malleable, withdrawn, dependant. Rennie was anything but that. I held my breath. But they took the chance. There was only one hitch; Rennie would have to be held for another ten days. Rennie's daughter was called in for respite. She took her mother home to Chico and lasted less than three days. She returned her to her brother and fled back to Chico. It was clear that Rennie couldn't be returned home to me alone, at least not yet. So her son held her for another hellish week. Then he delivered her to Farrell Crest and in relief, left her there.

In Farrell Crest, Rennie was even worse. She was now acutely paranoid. She was cruelly sarcastic, disruptive and quarrelsome. She even tried to lead a rebellion and exodus among the other patients. She telephoned every one she ever knew at all hours, all over the world, to tell them she was a prisoner in jail, and that I had put her there. Simultaneously, she called me...and called me...and called me. During one trip down to see her, she called and left a message on the machine 21 times.

Every day, for the entire day, I drove down to Farrell Crest and took Rennie out. Out to walk, out to play on the beach, out to fly a kite, out for coffee - anything at all that would get her out of the home and the paralyzing environment of somnolent Alzheimer's patients and the largest TV set I have ever seen. Each time Rennie would throw a hysterical tantrum, she was relentlessly paranoid. Why was I keeping her locked up? Give me the car keys NOW. The tantrum could and often did last all day. But I persisted and the idea for '*the Plan*' began to emerge.

By now I had come to know some people, done some research, found some alternatives. I located a neuropsychiatrist who I was sure would be perfect for Rennie. But there was a catch. Her practice was closed. I called in everyone who might swing some weight in the medical community and its periphery, even to prevailing on my daughter-in-law, a neurologist, to try to influence Dr. Feinstein to accept Rennie. I wrote imploring letters to her. If it would have helped, I would have begged on bended knee, without kneepads. And, bless her heart, one day she agreed to see Rennie during her day in the emergency room at French NPI. She spoke with her for over an hour…and agreed to take her case. I felt like sending her flowers.

Each day when I took Rennie out of Farrell Crest for our outing she would begin the endless litany, 'Why have you put me here? What have I done? I haven't committed a crime. Give me the keys to my car.' It often ran without pause, all day. Then when we returned, it would escalate, ending in an impressive tantrum outside the facility, where she would lock herself, arms and legs, to the car and refuse to get out, screaming and ranting. At such times, I walked a few yards away and waited. Once in a while she would calm down, but more often the director would have to come out and coax her indoors.

I persisted. I took her now to a theater matinee, another time to Chinese dinner, to the library, to a rock and mineral show. I scoured the papers for activities in reasonable distance of the Farrell Crest Facility. We went to lunch, we went to coffee shops, and we walked and walked and walked on the beach. Her behavior continued fierce enough to blister the paint on the car. Still…there were times she was almost conversational. The suicide threats continued. Once she even tried to jump out of the car while it was moving, but they were fewer. She began to offer thoughts such as, 'There is no point in my trying to escape… they'll only send someone after me and take me back.' It wasn't exactly good, but it was getting better. Yet Rennie continued to be fiercely disruptive, catastrophic and hysterical at the Farrell Crest Facility. The owners asked me not to come every day, that it was upsetting her, that she needed to accept this home as hers for the rest of her life. The very idea chilled me. For a few days I skipped an occasional day… then I resumed the daily commute and *the Plan*, which now was taking form and purpose. It was, in reality, little more than forced activity, exercise and mental stimulation. I had no reason to believe it would work, but I had tried everything else. The brain responds to stimulation, so my only hope in resurrecting it was to stimulate.

I brought kites to fly and games to play...Backgammon, Scrabble, Yahtzee. I brought her a camera to encourage her to see things beyond her trouble, books and poems to intrigue her mind. I wrote poems to her to enhance her feelings of self-worth and then asked her to help me improve them.

As I mentioned, Dr. Feinstein had accepted her case. I set about transferring her from the previous Psychiatrist, whom she truly hated. In securing her medical records from the office of the latter, I happened to glance through them and there on the last line of the last page was *it*.... finally. Diagnosis: ALZHEIMER'S

The very first time I had *ever seen* the diagnosis.

Rennie would not allow me in the office when she visited Dr. Feinstein. During those interviews she had always been rude, demanding, dissatisfied with everything happening. For the last five minutes I would be allowed in. Invariably it took at least that long to set the record straight, to correct the lies and distortions Rennie had fabricated. As soon as we left the office, without exception, Rennie would recall that the doctor, always a man, had spent the whole time talking with me and paid no attention to her at all. This happened even when I was out of the city. For the sake of balance in the appraisal and to keep her current on response to medication etc., I picked up the idea of keeping Dr. Feinstein current with faxed reports. I would send her a status and progress report before each monthly meeting.

What began to happen now, with the introduction of Dr. Feinstein into *the Plan*, was a whole new philosophy of treatment. If Rennie were much younger, say thirty or so, I suspect that she would have been diagnosed schizophrenic, probably paranoid though with strong compulsive obsessive overtones. Her paranoia was prominent and pervasive. So was depression. But she was eighty-one and the diagnosis is reflexive most of the time. My mother had died of senile dementia. It's a good thing she did it 45 years ago, otherwise, she would have had to go through Alzheimer's.

Well, as I knew, there is no treatment for Alzheimer's. It was pointless and frustrating to hope or search for help there. So, we began treating what we could see and changing proprietaries constantly as we watched for effects. Ativan for the agitation, Antidepressives for the depression and a neuroleptic (Moban) for the psychotic symptoms.

And things changed. Not right away. Not a lot. But they changed, and *the*

Plan continued. One promising sign was that Rennie became part of the 'microsociety' at Farrell Crest. She adopted her roommate, a childlike Alzheimer's case, and brought her little presents each time we returned to Farrell Crest from our outings. She took over chores, such as setting the table and washing the dishes. Then she began to participate in the care of the patients. If I know my Rennie, they had to exercise some firmness to keep her from taking charge altogether. But a significant aspect of this development was that they very apparently could actually trust her. It was becoming clear that Rennie was functioning on a level between the other patients and the professional staff, and my plan called for stimulation and encouragement in an environment more suited to her abilities and clarity. She could now be trusted closer to home, and the shorter commute would help us both. Alyce Hartford sent me to the Ombudsmen and to someone named Jerry. That was another pivotal moment. Jerry immediately appraised the situation accurately and recommended Ocean View in Cayucos.

Ocean View is a converted motel. It has entirely private rooms. Residents may bring their own furniture and favorite possessions. There is a large garden and gazebo, a spacious living room, kitchen and dining room, all in addition to the rooms, some of which are outdoors and some interior. More important, most of the residents are communicative, socially participatory and alert. And there is an atmosphere of freedom, self-determination and responsibility. Once settled in, residents may be permitted to walk alone around the adjacent blocks and may even walk unattended on the beach across the street. It is a really nice place, well run by a mother/daughter team of Rns. And there was a waiting list.

I left no rocks unturned trying to get Rennie at the head of the list as soon as possible. Friends like Alyce and Jerry provided recommendations. Dr. Feinstein called and reassured them that Rennie was suitable. But it still took weeks.

November 16th we moved Rennie to Ocean View. She was belligerent and depressed. She had believed she was going home. But there began a partnership with the very sympathetic, very capable owner, Lorraine. Lorraine kept an unobtrusive but keen and insightful watch over Rennie and reported to me her adjustment to the home, her alertness, her participation and her progress. And it was encouraging.

Meanwhile, the plan ground on. Now every day was occupied with activity, no time…no hours off. Everyday I took Rennie out. We walked the beaches, we had lunch at restaurants, and we went to the theater matinees and now, for the first time, we went out evenings. We went to evening theater, concerts and events that only happened at night. It all seemed to go very well, although not so much so to Rennie. Perhaps she just wanted to go home.

And one day, with my heart in my throat, I kept an appointment with Lorraine and asked the question for which I feared the answer; did she think Rennie might ever go home? She said, 'Certainly, when do you want to take her?' I was elated, overjoyed and frightened. We talked about it. I explained phase two of my plan and told her that I would like to have Rennie home for Christmas. However, I didn't want it to coincide with the day itself. I didn't want it to conflict with the effulgence of the occasion. I wanted it to happen enough before that, for her to be ready for Christmas, and in order to give us a chance to adjust and decorate before the day, and yet also I wanted it to have some symbolic significance. I selected the twenty-first, the Winter Solstice, the beginning of winter, the day of new beginnings.

Now with renewed hope, I visited Rennie and took her out of Ocean View. We would proceed in one single direction…south toward home. At first I took her to the beach in front of Ocean View and we walked southerly, not northerly as always before. The next day we would picnic at Morro Strand Beach, a mile or so farther south. Then we picnicked and walked the beach at San Jacinto. We shopped at Spencers Market, which then was called Giant Foods. Next day we walked the beach near Morro Rock. Then we visited the Community Center in Morro Bay. Then for several days we had our coffee at the Embarcadero and lunched in Morro Bay.

And one day we made a major step, the first moment in Los Osos. I took Rennie to the outdoor coffee shop at the Second Street pier in Baywood, where before, we had gone for coffee nearly every afternoon for years. It was a momentous occasion, seeing for the first time all her friends from the old life, facing her own fear and embarrassment, for now she was fully conscious that she had been ill, publicly and spectacularly ill, and there may be social fences to mend.

And so it inched. One momentous day we went home for an hour. Rennie tended some of her plants, then we returned to the coffee shop and back to Ocean View. By now, some of the clamor to go home had died down.

One fateful day she had said, 'I place myself entirely in your hands; I will do whatever you want.'

Now each time she had to return to Ocean View she accepted it as a step in the slow gradual process of returning home. She could see beyond the day…there was a future.

Gradually, ever so gradually, we would visit the house for longer periods, then return to coffee on 2nd Street as reinstatement of an old routine, and then back to Ocean View. One day I picked her up before breakfast, took her home for gardening, then to lunch, to the beach, to coffee, dinner at home, TV for a couple of hours and back to Ocean View. Without a seam, with no notice at all on her part, we had stayed at home for one whole day. The next morning I picked Rennie up again before breakfast. We spent the day together, had dinner at home, decorated the house a little, went to bed and slept the night. It was the 21st of December.

She has never left since."

Chapter Sixteen

Kind sleep steals away the weary course
Life's promise kept at last…

Tom's recounting of Rennie's Alzheimer's is poignant, and there is a major victory to be shared, one that not many of us could have hoped to achieve. There seems to be, indeed, a miraculous cure that took place. Tom is quick to point out that he has no scientific basis to believe that there is a method he pioneered that can be repeated. He had only one patient, and that patient was a special case. Yet it is impossible now to imagine that Rennie has ever been anything other than a bright, focused woman. She recalls the time herself. She reflects on it and agrees with the accounting. She has no explanations to offer; of course, only that she confirms Tom's remarks.

To this day, she remains a viable woman within the realm of normalcy considering her advancing years.

The details of Tom and Rennie's lives were disclosed to a select few. It remains a mystery as to the miracle that transformed Rennie, yet the community suspects that there was a combination of events that led to her recovery. Most believe that there was a unique application of love and science, and as a result there may be hope for others facing similar tragedy. It remains an unbelievable accounting, yet the events stand.

At a final taping session with Tom and Rennie, final questions were asked.

"Tom, when you brought Rennie home for the final time, did you know then that it was over? Did you think she would be home to stay?"

Tom smiled and said, "I have to backtrack a little. It was not so clean and simple as all that, so no, I wasn't absolutely sure. I keep a logbook. There is an entry in it from when things were darkest, when it was clear at that time, that Rennie would never get well, and all I wanted in my life was to have her back. It was a night when, through tears in my eyes, I wrote, 'this is going to break my heart.' Later that same night January 29th, I had a heart attack. It was a third degree block.

911 brought the emergency team and the ambulance, and I nearly didn't make it. There is no doubt in anyone's mind that the distal cause was stress, pure and simple and extreme.

Immediate surgery was required, but I wouldn't allow it at that time. Rennie couldn't be left alone. Someone had to stay with her, someone had to be found. And two days later there was a crucial appointment with Dr. Feinstein, one in which treatment and medication plans were to be readjusted for the long haul back in the real world. So early that morning I left the hospital, arranged familiar help for Rennie, went to the appointment with Dr. Feinstein and called the cardiologist to say, 'OK, now.'

Following that incident, I was able to recuperate, but when I finally brought Rennie home, I still suffered chest pains, and wasn't certain of either of two things; the first, if she would be permanently home, the second, if I would live to see it regardless."

"So… you were suffering from your *own* health problems through all of this?"

"Oh yes," Tom answered, "Yes, and there were many. I may not have mentioned it, but there was an incident that happened to me which may have led, inadvertently to the 'cure' for Rennie. Near the beginning of all this, I started to suffer from chronic pain. I didn't know the cause, and after many failed attempts at diagnosis, including attempts to pass it off as arthritis, I realized that I had Fibromyalgia. It's a condition that's usually misdiagnosed, and frequently the physician gives up and recommends a psychiatrist. It's a condition that has no known cause or treatment, yet it's crippling. It will mimic the symptoms of arthritis, but it takes over your entire body, all at once.

There came a point at which I could hardly walk across the room, even with my crutches, and ultimately I was referred to a counselor. I knew it was not a mental condition, I'm in a position to know these things, yet there was no relief in sight. At some point, in desperation, I saw a chiropractor in Morro Bay named Dr. Wilkins. I was amazed, he not only diagnosed the disease, he was conversant with the 'eleven trigger points' that are essential in diagnosis.

Dr. Wilkins immediately pressed on a point, and it nearly sent me through the roof. This doctor was honest enough to tell me that he didn't know of any cure, but I was able to take the information to my physician, who was forced to reconsider his diagnosis. Yet still, he had no suggestions by way of relief. I was referred, eventually, to a medical school in Arizona. The Medical Director himself saw me and gave validation. The director asked if he could bring in several students, and I agreed to it.

Once the students were assembled, the Director left them, but instructed them each to arrive at a diagnosis. When he returned, he questioned them individually in front of me. 'What does he have?' he asked the first student.

'Arthritis,' the student replied.

'What does he have?' he asked the second student.

'Arthritis,' was the second reply, and so it went for all of them.

The Director then reached over my back and pressed on a certain point, sending me into agonizing pain. 'Do you think that particular point has anything to do with arthritis?' the Director asked.

'No,' Came the groups' response.

'You must *learn*...' the Director continued, 'to diagnose Fibromyalgia.' So, I had my diagnosis, but it left me helpless and hopeless. There is, and was, no cure. But, after I returned home, a dear friend of mine who was aware of my condition came to visit. Ray asked me if I would go on a drive with him, and I agreed. We ended up in Montana de Oro State park. It was a beautiful day and I enjoyed the drive and the company, but when we reached the end of the road, Ray asked me if I would like to take a short walk. I told him that it was impossible for me and since he knew how much pain walking caused, it irritated me that he would even ask. But Ray persisted. He asked me if I would just walk a few paces ... there was something that he wanted to show me. I did and it hurt, but Ray kept me occupied in conversation so I was distracted for a while. At one point, Ray suddenly stopped and made me look up. To my surprise, I had walked nearly fifty yards! There was a spectacular view of the ocean, and I remember thinking, that if I could make it that far, once, I could do it again, so I resolved to walk every day.

I decided to quantify it and to push myself a little further each day, so in order to make that easy, I drove to the pier in Cayucos, and started.

The first day I only made it about 30 feet before I stopped and turned around. It was hard going on crutches as the weathered boards were irregular and had large cracks. Plus, I didn't have Ray to distract me from the pain. But I was proud of the accomplishment regardless, and on the next day I added a few feet.

After several months, I finally made it to the end of the pier. As I stood there looking down at the dark water, I contemplated the crutches for a moment, and then on impulse I heaved them into the ocean. Now, I realized, I was stuck. If I wanted to go home, I would have to walk back to the car without crutches.

It was a long journey back to the car, I can assure you, but by the time I made it there. I knew I would conquer this disease. From that point forward, I walked every day, until I was up to several miles.

Somewhere along the way, the pain stopped and was gone forever. I'm not sure how or why this worked, but I literally walked the disease away."

"So…Tom, what do you think this had to do with Rennie and Alzheimer's?"

"Oh yes!" Tom said, "I nearly forgot the point. I'm thinking, and this has no basis in science, that the stimulation of Rennie's brain worked in the same way as the forced stimulation on my body. There is no way to know if this is true or not. There are no studies. I no longer have a lab, a forum, colleagues, a university and a library, grants, nor access to them. I mention it to anyone who will listen, but in this milieu of treatment and care, I'm dealing only with clinicians, nurses and doctors. I suspect they are secretly amused at my obsession with causes but not much interested."

"But your 'treatment' for her has been mental stimulation?"

"Among other things, yes," Tom answers, "I keep her on a healthy diet as a minimum, don't I, Wren?" Tom asks Rennie.

"Yes," she says, "He won't let me have any of the things I like." She finishes with a smile.

"What, exactly, are you both eating?"

"For the most part, I keep Rennie on three healthy meals a day. Grains and from five to twenty different vegetables daily, along with soy milk, juices, fruit, seafood. I run a regular health farm here. But the most important 'treatment' is her walks with Minnie and me. We walk and swim, and I reward her with a trip to a Jacuzzi at the end of a particularly hard day. It is all about stimulation, both mental and physical. We go to the theater, lectures, support groups and movies. I take her everywhere. We still go to coffee, and all I can say is, that this worked. I don't necessarily know how, I didn't know what I was doing at the time, but it worked.

You see, fate is relentless, but I don't believe the brain just one day gives up, gets tired of working and sets about destroying itself. There are no cases of 'remission' that I'm aware of and yet, here we are. This is unusual. This has never happened before. It's unheard of. No physician, or scientist, no worker in Alzheimer's disease has ever heard of it happening before. One in a thousand patients go through violent behavior and inevitably into phase III and death.

Violent behavior in itself is extremely rare and recovery is never. And I must caution that even if it were possible to snatch someone from that agony as I have done, you would have to be able to devote every moment of the rest of your life, every thought, every plan, every detail, forsaking everything else – as I have done.

All that must be done, all that, all the stress, pain and loss of meaning in life, all for the off chance, the extremely unlikely long shot, all is done for the sake of being able to stay the inevitable for a while. I tell you and I tell everyone, that I'm telling my story only to illustrate one single point; never, never give up. Never stop hoping.

No one is sure what really can be done or what might happen. And then I tell them an anecdote. For a very long time, each time I saw Rennie in the home, after she stormed and raved for an hour or so, she would ask me please, please to help her die. We had talked about this before, how neither of us wanted to live as a burden, as a vegetable, or extend a life in which there was no joy or hope of it. We had filed and distributed power of attorney for health decisions long ago, made funeral arrangements, a trust, all the responsible thoughtful moves.

She had a point. It's what I would want certainly, I would not want to live with agony such as hers. How could I let her suffer so? I could easily have helped her out of life and compassion, care and love told me I should. But I couldn't. No heroism, no minute excavation of conscience, no philosophical debate. I couldn't. So, I did what I could do. I kept on keeping on.

And then one day she emerged lucid, smiling, buoyant, manageable, cooperative and.... most of all, happy. And, if I had helped her die, however honorable or compassionate it might have been...we would have missed these wonderful years together. So *no*. Don't ever give up hope. Don't hope for the impossible. Just don't give up and the *possible* may very well happen and be all you could hope for.

We have each other still. We will hug and hold hands and walk the little Corgi, Minnie, and have Coffee on 2nd Street...

Tom's poem to Rennie----published by Taproot Press in the book
The Long Good Night – poems by Tom Law.

Now that it is over and the chance is gone,
Have I done it all?
Have I done it well? Well enough, all along?

I meant to say I love you all the times I should,
All the drear sad times you needed that to hold –
Not half as much as I planned to say,
Nor a hundredth what would keep at bay
The deranged dragons in the dark for one more night.

I hope you sensed the fineness though
In a passing touch, in love tucked among the morning strawberries;
In the intimacy of pillows,
The watchful eagerness of words, the questions that scaffold my concern
And swept past the door the terror dogs.
I meant to fold you into comfort, blanket warmth,
Sleepy snuggles, for the child you never got to be.

When I felt the shrinking days
I like to think I captured some crackles of the light
To measure out to you each evening in luminous fragments
Like metaphysical fireflies.
Can you forgive me if sometimes it was all I could do
To keep you safe one more time?
Sometimes it seemed the whole of life
Was just not dying.
All I might have done groans in the wind now
And blows away,
Whispers of adieu.

If I could not bear to part with the storm of you
How much should I have mourned each raindrop
As it fell away?
Which drop dissolved the cherished you of you?

Couldn't you tell me when you were not there?
The principle that plucked us from the pond
Shaped your breast to fit my hand
As sweet wine seamless fills the glass.
It seems at last the wine is emptied out,

And I must sweep away
The broken glass of memories,

And let you go to drift apart
Beyond the solemn curve of day,
Carefree on puffs of cloud,
Old men's long white beards
Tucked into the collar of the horizon,
Wafting you home.

You're safe beyond the reach of love or fright,
Sheltered in the farthest cave of sleep
Where populations of the past await your dreams
To come to life again.

It would betray all we have been
Not to loose your hand and let you go but
What shall I do now
With all this useless love?

Dr. Tom, Rennie and their little Corgi, Minnie, live peacefully in Los Osos. Rennie continues to be active in the early Alzheimer's group, which she, along with Tom's help, founded many years ago. Her health is maintained.

Dr. Tom surprises Rennie each and every important holiday with a local choral group who serenades her with love songs and gives her flowers. A playful enactment and testimony to their continued love for each other. These celebrations are also enjoyed by their many friends and associates.

They still enjoy Coffee on 2nd Street, holding hands and watching sunsets over the sand dunes.

243

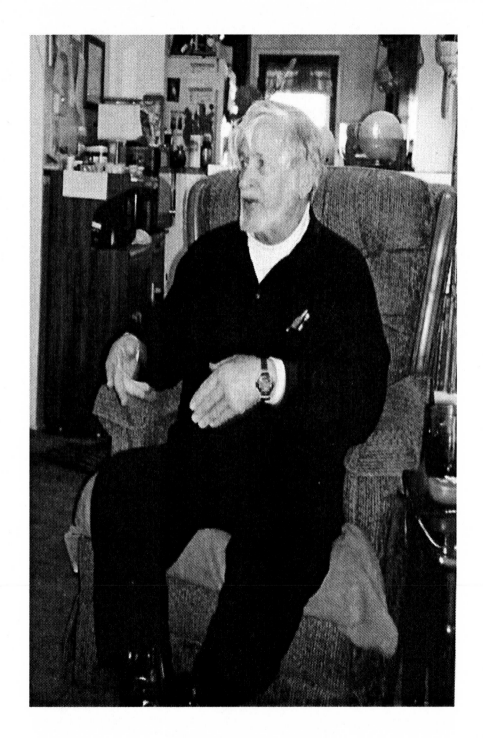

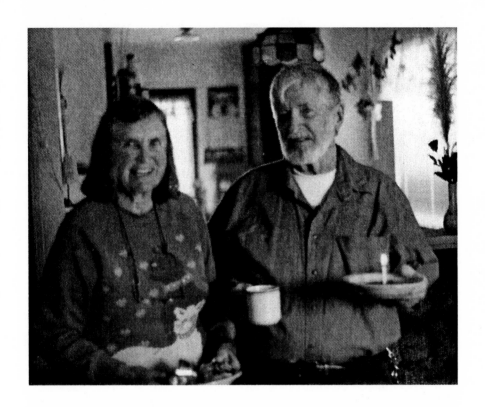

While this is a biography and true, the various names of doctors and persons and places have, for the most part, been changed to respect their privacy.

Epilogue

Tom sat beside me in his driveway on a small chair. In front of us was the new, "Ural" motorcycle that he had recently purchased, solely for the purpose of taking Rennie on afternoon excursions. It had to be a Ural, since that was one of the only companies around that made new motorcycles with a sidecar. The old Suzuki Savage sat nearby. Tom had discovered, in his last trip with Rennie, that leaning a motorcycle as you do going around a curve really disturbed her, yet she loved the open air. Some of her 'free spirit' returned and was visible in her smile with the wind blowing across her face once again. She was no longer able to manage a motorcycle on her own, so the compromise was to be the sidecar.

I tinkered with the drive shaft and took advantage of the opportunity to ask questions of Tom. There was nothing wrong with the drive shaft, but I felt if I tinkered long enough, I could hold his attention.

"OK," I said, as I wiped away an imaginary spot of grease, "I sent an excerpt of an email that you had sent me to a lady friend, and she was quite perturbed over it."

"Oh Gawd," Tom groaned, "What did it say?"

"Oh, I think it was an answer to one of my questions regarding marriage, and the comments you had made regarding it," I said.

"Aiiiieee! Pobrecita!!" Tom exclaimed, lapsing into Spanish, "These are the very things you must be careful with, Steve, if you want to keep your lady friend around! Remember, you need to assure her that these are the programs built in around the ice age. They go on running whether we need them or not. We just have to be on our guard and not let the dogs slip the leash, remember? I said none of this applies to present company. We are not acquiring these genetic programs now nor necessarily allowing them to run, though they will run if left untended. These things are likely to underlie much of our behavior to the extent we allow it, but they do not, by any means, still *necessarily* determine it."

I laughed and knew it was true, but it was just that I had often wondered

246

about the convention of marriage and Tom had answered, dutifully, from his scientific perspective. He had actually answered my question with another question, regarding the historic significance of the bride being a virgin and followed that with the observation that there were stringent social implications around pre-marital sex.

I had given up on the answer and Tom provided it for me. He had said, "There is always the possible answer that restricted sexual activity, in the extreme case, virginity, is an effective way to combat sexually transmitted diseases. However, if that were a valid argument, why is virginity and fidelity imposed almost totally on the female?"

"Also," Tom continued, "I believe we may safely assume that sexual transmission of disease greatly antedated knowledge of how it happened. And cultural imposition of female virginity is as old as history."

"OK," I said, "Then why the obsession with it?"

"Reproductive strategy," Tom said, "For the male. How much compensation is he willing to accept to abandon his patently efficient horny rabbit strategy?"

"You mean," I said, "The inherent strategy of males to mate wherever and whenever they get a chance?"

"Exactly," Tom said, "The male is giving up a lot of potential here by committing to a single female. When in reality if there were no social restrictions, he could potentially father hundreds of children. Yet, he is called upon to accept dedication of all his reproductive energy to one female, one nest."

"But that's what the *female* has to do, so isn't it only fair that the male should as well!" I objected.

"Fairness is not a part of the equation in the battle of the sexes," Tom said, "It's all about strategies. A female can only give birth to one child a year, so she is much more limited. The male is really holding back his reproductive potential by denying himself other females."

"OK," I said, "Then tell me. Why does he do it?"

Tom watched as I checked the oil on the motorcycle for the third time. I was not paying attention to what I was doing, but he didn't seem to mind. He continued with his answer, "The male accepts the tradeoff *especially* because humans *particularly* have a postnatal development period of many years. A bunny strategy is appropriate in species in which there is no, or virtually no, postnatal development period requiring parental care. In most of those species the young are born capable of motility and self-feeding. The absence of parental care is offset by a high birth rate and a high mortality rate. Most of them get eaten. So the *human* male stays in the vicinity of the mother of his children in order to participate to some extent in protecting and nourishing them. If this is not his strategy, at least until the children reach puberty, then the probability of survival to reproductive age of the young is reduced. In fact the longer, postnatally, the father hangs around, the greater his investment, but also it offsets the waste that would occur if his children died from lack of his protection.

Conversely, the sacrifice of dissemination of his genes over a wider population of females with a greater number of progeny is an irretrievable asset. It becomes of overwhelming importance to make the sacrifice count, to see his kids survive."

"So," I said, "The male sticks around to raise his children, and that's why he is 'willing' to commit."

"Yes," Tom replied.

"But what about your comments on chastity and virginity, how is that a part of the formula?" I asked.

Tom smiled, "Well, in order for the male to allocate all of his energies to a single female and her young, he must make *darn* sure that they are *his* kids. If he is fooled into raising children not genetically related, he has wasted the children he could have had by a bounding habit and not realized those he should have had at maturity in compensation for his sacrifice. Hence sequestering the female from other males becomes important, second to nothing less than impregnation itself. And you can see why we have chastity belts. And in *their* absence, cultural 'virtual' chastity belts such as patriarchal marriage, virginity at marriage, 'commitment' and 'relationships' and so on."

I thought about this for a while, and once again marveled that the facts fit the observations. It did serve, however, to ruin some of the romance.

"So that's the bit on marriage," I said.

"Biologically speaking," Tom said.

I set a wrench down and leaned back in the sun. It was a beautiful afternoon, and the cool air from the ocean was just enough to keep the pavement of the driveway from getting too hot. I heard the front door of Toms house open, and Rennie walked out, trailing their corgi, Minnie.

"Hello, dear," Tom said.

"Hello," Rennie said, "What are you boys doing?"

"Working on the bike," Tom answered.

"When will it be ready?" Rennie asked.

Tom looked at me and I said, "It's ready now, Rennie, but I'm just checking it over."

Rennie smiled, and continued down the street with Minnie. Tom watched her as she went.

"So, Tom," I said, not quite finished with the discussion, "When *you* gave up your 'free-ranging' male drives to be with Rennie, it could not have been for the purpose of making sure your children survived. You were fifty and she was sixty. What made you decide to marry?"

Tom tore his gaze away from Rennie and looked back at me. He thought for a moment then said, "There is the other side of the contract. The advantages of free-ranging masculinity, not to mention the pleasures, have an overwhelming appeal, biologically, evolutionarily, psychologically and personally. Alas, there are losses in any compromise. But remember we weren't meant to live beyond 25 to 40 years at most, prior to the advances in the modern era. Being old is a state not selected for in evolution. In a very real sense, in that consummation, we are very much on our own.

What I value most now is twofold: one can be summarized in the poem "Tandem" I wrote not long ago; the other can be summarized by the entire poetry book.

They are, in essence, the catalog of shared memories. A higher order interaction, or in other words, the whole is greater than the sum of the parts. It is a united front toward life, the feeling of us against them, a feeling of unspoken trust and confidence and being able to depend on the known conduct of another in a pinch. These are the things you start to value as you go through life.

The heart of the poetry book I wrote for Rennie is, or should be, that there is an unspoken wholeness to the two of us. Sometimes it is as simple as a comfortable bed in which to lie down and die, and knowing that you have spent your time with a person you love and cherish. Frankly, Steve, I wouldn't trade that for all the babes on 'Baywatch.' The choice for the last quarter century, to do it all over again, would be the very same one that I made."

Tom was watching Rennie, who was down the road a short distance. It was easy to see how very much he loved her, and in spite of all the challenges he had faced, all the grim times, he was still happy to have her in his life. He was content with the choices he had made.

"So it changes with age?" I asked.

"Oh yes," Tom said, "It changes a lot. As we grow older we're faced with the stark reality that we do not fit the esthetic ideal any longer. But keep this in perspective, there is no intrinsic beauty in youth. It's programmed into us to value youth just for the reasons I mentioned, but beauty is in the *perception* of it. I find Rennie beautiful, and I cannot explain why. She just is."

I could see that Tom was totally in love with Rennie. Still, even after all these years. She was frail and needed his constant attention, but she was his mate for life. There was a bond between them that defied description; a deep uniting force that held them together through everything, yet still allowed just enough apartness, that individuality we must posses, to be the assurance for a fulfillment of life together. It was a link that made each of their lives complete. Tom had always been open and honest with me. He held nothing back in his discussions. Each question I asked, over the years, was answered directly, completely and without reservations. I had become deeply reliant on this source of information. It was clear that he had resolved his life in terms of relationships. His example of love and adoration belied the fact that no amount of genetic or evolutionary programming could control him. He was free to love completely.

But I still wondered about the future of mankind. The past was fairly clear now. The journey we had taken to arrive at this point. But I wondered, where were we going?

I could see that Tom was getting ready to call it a day, but I ventured one last question. "If we have these programs running, in the most basic and fundamental parts of our brains, yet now, having become aware of them and realizing that they may not serve our purposes today, in the modern era, how do you see us changing in the future? Will we change? Or will we continue as hapless pawns of genetics?"

Tom laughed, "No one has a crystal ball, Steve, but there is, I suppose, a new awareness growing. We are probably the only living organism that knows it's going to die from the beginning of our lives. That makes all the difference. That's all that matters. Being the sole form of life aware of our genetic destiny, we are also the only animal with the possibility of changing it. We may fail that chance, but it's there.

That we have the potential to change ourselves removes us from the exclusive grasp of *pure* chance for the first time. What we do, or even *if* we do, and including the excellent possibility that we'll blow it, is secondary to the fact that we *can* make a change.

The evolution of life takes a long-term perspective. Extremely long. One small bump in the chronicle of a species is a singular event in what often takes millions of years. The first rocket, maybe even the first propellant, was that lump. To the future of humans it may well offer the transformation similar to another lump that was the beginning of a wing, thus giving flight to birds. It may, of course, also be the lump that proves fatal to the species.

But first we have that lump, and second and even more important, we have the capacity to encourage, pursue, develop and exploit it. Does any bird know it has a crest and wear a diadem on it? Is there a peacock yet that has developed a tail enhancing cosmetic industry?

We are the only living thing that is aware of traits and features, and we manipulate them. We know of our genetic composition, our inherited destiny and we are directing it, consciously altering the very nature of tomorrow.

The very phrase 'genetic engineering' holds all the hope we need. All the forces of darkness, the devils that would keep us imprisoned slaves of our inherited biology are constantly at war with the forces that would redirect human nature toward its higher, more admirable, potential.

So, contrary to being 'victims' of genetics, we are the first life form, and maybe the last on this earth with the opportunity to free ourselves from it, to use it to form a destiny of our own. We hold our future in the palm of our hands. Maybe genetics sets the limits. But maybe that is only the architecture, not the furniture. Our genetic inventory is enormous, and we have only just begun to tap the resources. We do not yet realize our full potential, and if we make some wrong choices, we probably never will. Yet, through it all, we have the chance. It is a gift we should not take lightly. Look up, Steve; there are human footprints on the moon. They are there to remind us of what we can be."

Tom finished, and I could see he was tired. I thanked him for his time, and he rose and slowly ambled toward the small cottage that he and Rennie had shared for years. Rennie was just returning from walking Minnie, and she met Tom as he got up from his chair. Their hands met, and they slowly made their way to the front door. Tom looked back, and after guiding his beloved wife inside, gave a short wave to me and closed the door behind him.

From the Poem Tandem

...it was a honeymoon that left an impression.
After that the Herreshoff sloop
and the great timbered ketch,
the too wide seas and the snarling storms.
Two on the hammering deck in a raging battle
to wrench the cloth from the blunt demon claws.
Nothing to see through the bullet rain – no time to fear
Voiceless in the menace of the banshee blast,
room for just one thought: sail out or drown.
Then lift, swift as a plane,
to the dragon teeth of a tidal bore,
flung high up on the window of water
and over and alive
and they did sail home.

And so went the cycle,
feet tracing the sine of the years pedaling on,
the panorama just out of view,
the sea, the trees, the yawning road-
a thought, no more;
a snap to be viewed at home, at rest
as she pumped and furled and leaned and tended,
eyes locked to the deck the road the task at her feet,
just getting the two of them home
one more time.

It's the bottom of the hill, love.
Rest now.

O. Thomas Law
Born: July 9, 1925
Children: Twin sons, 1954

EDUCATION

Bridgeport High School, Bridgeport, West Virginia   1939-1943
University of Hawaii, Honolulu   1945-1946
West Virginia University, Morgantown   1946-1947
University of Michigan, Ann Arbor   1947-1949 B.A.
                                                                                        1949-1950 M.A.
                                                                                        1950-1952 Ph.D.
Johns Hopkins University, Baltimore, Post-Doctoral Fellow 1952-1954
Oregon State University, Electronics   1965
Duke University, Senior Post-Doctoral Fellow   1967-1968

PROFESSIONAL EXPERIENCE

University of Michigan, Teaching Fellow   1949-1951
Vision Research Lab. University of Michigan, Research   1951-1952
National Science Foundation, U.S. Public Health Service 1952-1954
Post-Doctoral Fellow, Johns Hopkins University   1952-1954
Vision Research Lab, University of Michigan, Research   1954-1956
Mental Health Research Institute, University of Michigan,
Director of Electrophysiological Laboratories   1956-1960
University of Michigan, Psychology Department,
Lecturer in Psychology   1959-1960
Autonetics Corp., Downey, Calif., Senior Research Engr.   1960-1961
Claremont Graduate School, Associate Professor   1961-1963
Professor   1963
Duke University, Durham, North Carolina, Senior
Post-Doctoral Fellow, Neuroscience Program   1967-1968

OTHER EXPERIENCE

Consultant in Neurophysiology and polygraphy, Michigan
Joint Schizophrenia Research Project, Ypsilanti State Hospital 1958-1960
Consultant in Vision, Electro Optical Systems   1965
Consultant in Psychophysiology, Beckman Instruments   1966
Expert Witness, Visual Parameters and Properties   continuous
Consultant in Biofeedback, Inland Psychiatric Medical Group   1973-

PERSONAL ACTIVITIES

Editor, Neuroscience's Abstracts   1967-
Reviewing Editor, Science   1959-

GRANTS AND AWARDS

Fellows of the University, Johns Hopkins University, (NIMH: 1952-53)

Principal Investigator U.S.P.H.S. Neural Mechanisms of Reproduction, University of Michigan, 1956

Principal Investigator, National Academy of Sciences, National Research Council (Committee for Research in Problems of Sex) Grant, Neurology of Emotion, University of Michigan, 1958-61)

Principal Investigator, U.S.P.H.S. (NIMH), Neural Mechanisms of Reproduction Grant, 1962, Supplementary Grant, 1962; Grant, 1963: Grant, 1964, Claremont Graduate School

Principal Investigator, Hancock Foundation Grant, Microelectrode Studies of the Neural Mechanisms of Sexual Behavior, Claremont Graduate School, 1965, 1966, 1967

Senior Post-doctoral Fellow, Duke University, Neuroscience Program, 1967-68

Principal Investigator, Claremont Graduate School Faculty Grants, 1968

Principal Investigator, NIMH Grant, Evoked Limbic Unit Response to Stimulation, 1969-70

GRANTS APPLIED FOR;

1972 - 1973
5-2-73 "Human Infertility via Conditioned Hyperthermia." Graduate Research Committee.
5-2-73 "Vaginal pH and Ovulation." Graduate School Research Committee.
5-2-74 "Visible Neuron Frequencies." Graduate School Research Committee.
5-2-73 "The Effects of Exogenously & Endogenously Induced Scrotal Hyperthermia in the Rat." Internal Research Grant.

5-3-73 "The Effects of Exogenously & Endogenously Induced Scrotal Hyperthermis in the Rat." SPSSI, Department of Psychology, Michigan State University.

HONORS

Two graduate students have won the Young Psychologist Triennial Award of the American Psychological Association, 1966, 1969.
Honored Scholar, Colloquium of Scholars, California Lutheran College, 1973

HONORARY SOCIETIES

Phi Beta Kappa
Phi Kappa Phi
Phi Sigma (Biology)
Sigma Xi

OFFICES AND COMMITTEES

Past President, Sigma Xi Club, Claremont
Academic Procedures Committee
Research Committee (Faculty Research Grants)
Animal Care Committee
Equipment and Facilities Committee
Building Committee
Admissions Committee in Psychology

PROFESSIONAL SOCIETIES

American Physiological Society
American Association for the Advancement of Science
Medical Research Association of California
Psychonomic society
Western Psychological Association
West Coast Society for the Scientific Study of Sex
Federation of American Scientists in Experimental Biology
International Oceanographic Foundation

BIOGRAPHIES

Leaders in American Science
Who's Who in American Education
American Men and Women of Science
Who's Who in the West
National Register of Scientific Personnel
National Register of Prominent Americans and International Notables

TEACHING EXPERIENCE

Comparative Behavior and Evolution: Claremont Graduate School
Experimental Psychology, lecture and laboratory: University of Michigan
Physiological Psychology, lecture and laboratory: University of Michigan
  Claremont Graduate School
Neural Mechanisms of Behavior: University of Michigan
Sensory Physiology and Psychology: Claremont Graduate School
Electronics for Behavioral Scientists: University of Michigan
Physiological Measurements
Current Literature in Scientific Psychology: Claremont Graduate School
Methods and Techniques for the Study of the Nervous System: University
of Michigan
Neurophysiology of Emotion: University of Michigan Medical School
Properties of Dendrites: University of Michigan Medical School
Research in Physiological Psychology: Claremont Graduate School
Seminar in Teaching of Psychology: Claremont Graduate School
Evolution of the Mind and Brain: Claremont Graduate School
Comparative Behavior: Claremont Graduate School
Comparative Neuroanatomy: Claremont Graduate School
Advanced Physiological Psychology: California State University, Los
Angeles
Motivation and Emotion: Claremont Graduate School
Sex Behavior and Biology: Claremont Graduate School

ARTICLES & PUBLICATIONS

A two-factor theory of learning, M.A. thesis, University of Michigan, 1950

The effect of background luminance on brightness discrimination, Ph.D. Dissertation, University of Michigan, 1952

With Blackwell, J. R. White light photosensitization, J. Opt. Soc. Amer., 1953, 43

Preference in the rat for vertical and horizontal stripes after training on black-white discrimination. Amer. J. Psychol., 1954, 67, 714-716

With DeValois, R. The electrical threshold of the eye as a function of intensity and color of pre-adaptation. Amer. Psychol., 1955, 8

With DeValois, R. The electrical threshold of the eye as a function of frequency of stimulation. Amer. Psychol., 1955, 8

With DeValois, R. and Eliot. Electrical and optical indications of micro-fluctuations of the eye. Proj. Mich. Rep., 1955

With DeValois, R. Studies of the alleged electrosensitization of night vision. Proj. Mich. Rep., No. 2144-56-T, 1955

With DuValois, R. Eye position indication by means of the corneoretinal potential. Proj. Mich. Rep., No. 2144-56-T., 1956

With DuValois, R. Some results from electrical stimulation of the eye. First National Biophysics Conference, Columbus, Ohio, March 5, 1957, Reprint No. 5

With DeValois, R. Periorbital potentials recorded during small eye movements. Pap. Mich. Acad. Sci. Arts Lett., 1958, 43, 171-180

With Karinen, P. Effects of subcortical stimulation on sexual behavior in the male and female rat. Amer. Psychol., 1958, 13, 408 (Abstract)

With Meagher, W. Hypothalamic lesions and sexual behavior in the female rat. Science, 1958, 128, 1626-1627

With Wise, H.W. A multiple electrode carrier for chronic implantation in small animals. EEG Clin. Neurophysiol., 1958, 10, 749-751

With Greening. Human factors analysis of the field artillery digital automatic computer. Autonetics. TM 3041-93-23, 1960

A study of Minuteman maintenance problems as recorded in AMR system test logs. Autonetics, TM 3041-93-27, 1960

Polygraphy-measure of your emotions. Electronics Illus., 1960, 3,56,57, 111 with Gollander, M. and Isaacson, R.

Changes in circulating eosinophil levels associated with learned fear: Conditioned eosinopenia. J. Comp. Physiol. Psychol., 1960, 53, 520-523

With Karinen, P. Cardiac changes accompanying coitus in rats. J. Comp. Physiol. Psychol., 1961

With Adams, J. A versatile solderless electrode carrier for small animals. Psychol. Rep., 1963, 13, 539-541

With Skinner, J. E. Sexual behavior: Postcopulatory heart rate in the male and female rat. Psychon. Sci., 1964, 1, 235-236

With Watanabe, K. Techniques for chronic electrode implantation and brain potential recordings. Psychol. Rep., 1964, 15, 691-694

With Sackett, G.P. Hypothalamic potentials in the female rat evoked by hormones and by vaginal stimulation. Neuroendocrinology, 1966, 1, 31-44

With Rodgers, C. The effects of habenular and medial forebrain bundle lesions on sexual behavior in female rats. Psychon. Sci., 1967

With Gerbrandt, Lauren K. Sexual preference in female rats: I, II, Choices in tests with copulation. Psychon. Sci., 1967, Vol. 8 (11)

With Rodgers, C. H. Effects of chemical stimulation of the "limbic system" on lordosis in female rats. Physiol. Behav., Vol. 3, 241-246, 1968

With Moss, R. L. Influence of the estrous cycle on single cell activity in the forebrain. Brain Research, 1971, 23

With Moss, R. L. Response patterns of single cells in the forebrain to sexual stimuli. Brain Research, 1971, 23

With Paloutzian, R. and Moss, R. L. Effects of electrical stimulation of forebrain structures on copulatory behavior of ovariectomized, hormonetreated rats. Physiol. And Beh., 1971, 6

With French, D.J. and Fitzpatrick, D. Operant investigation of mating preference in female rats. J. of Comp. & Physiol. Psychol., 1972, Vol. 81, No. 2, 226-232

With Moss, R. L. and Paloutzian, R. Effects of electrochemical stimulation of forebrain structures on copulatory and stimulus bound in ovariectomized, hormone-treated rats. Physiol. and Behav., 1972

With French, D.J. & LeGare, Miriam. Single unit activity of convergent cells in the basal forebrain. Psychological Reports, 1972

With LeGare, Miriam & French, D.J. Single unit investigation of multiple modality systems and convergent cells in the hypothalamus. Submitted to Brain Research, 1973

With French, D.J. Leeb, C.S., Fahrion, S.L. and Jecht, E.W. Self-induced scrotal hyperthermia in man followed by decrease in sperm output: a preliminary report. Submitted to Science, January, 1973

With Wilsoncroft, W. Laboratory Manual of Physiological Psychology. Psychonomic Press, 1967

FILM

Searching the Brain. NBC-TV network. 1962

REPORTS, SYMPOSIA AND INVITED ADDRESSES

With O'Malley. The dependence of sexual behavior on basal diencephalic structures in the female rat. Symposium on "Progress in Physiological Psychology," American Psychological Association, 1957.

With Gollender and Isaacson. Conditioned eosinopenia. Eastern Psychological Association, Atlantic City, March, 1959.

With Gollender. Eosinopenia and limbic lesions. Eastern Psychological Association, New York, 1960.

Changes in heart rate in male and female rats during coitus. Midwestern Psychological Association, St. Louis, 1960.

With Adams, J. Brain mechanisms in sequential sexual behavior in male rats. Western Psychological Association, April, 1962.

With Skinner, J. E. Postcopulatory heart rate of the rat: A measure of central motivational states. Western Psychological Association, April, 1962.

With Adams, J. Brain mechanisms of sexual behavior in the male rat. California State Psychological Association, December, 1962.

With Forney, R. L. Consolidation of the memory trace. California State Psychological Association, December, 1962.

With Rodgers, C. H. Motivated vs. reflexive sexual behavior in the female rat. California State Psychological Association, December, 1962.

With Skinner, J. E. The effects of amygdalectomy on rats timulated in infancy. California State Psychological Association, December, 1962.

With Wilsoncroft, W. Maternal behavior in the rat. California State Psychological Association, December, 1962.

Chairman, Symposium, "Neurological research, perception, and reading." Claremont Reading Conference, February, 1963.

With Adams, J. Effects of subcortical lesions on sexual behavior in the male rat. Western Psychological Association, April, 1963.

With Forney, R. L. Retroactive effects of spreading depression. Western Psychological Association, April, 1963.

Chairman, Section in Physiology of Sexual Behavior, Western Psychological Association, April, 1963.

With Rodgers, C. H. Spontaneous and evoked sexual behavior in the female rat. A report on method of measurement and a study of the effects of subcortical lesions. Western Psychological Association, April, 1963.

With Watanabe, K. Subcortical EEG associated with reproductive behavior in the rat. Western Psychological Association, April, 1963.

With Wilsoncroft, W. Effect of median cortex lesions on maternal behavior in the rat. Western Psychological Association, April, 1963.

With Sackett, G. Hypothalamic potentials in the female rat evoked by hormones and by vaginal stimulation: Preliminary report. Western Psychological Association, April 1964.

With Watanabe, K. Subcortical EEG during mating in the female rat: Results of estrogen, progesterone, and sexual stimulation. Western Psychological Association, April, 1964.

Chairman, Section on Brain Mechanisms, Western Psychological Association, April, 1964.

Invited Address, Western Psychological Association, 1965. Neural mechanisms of sexual behavior.

With Gerbrandt, L. & Moss, R. Changes in response character of single hypothalamic cells to sensory and hormonal stimuli. West Coast Sex Conference, Palo Alto, 1966.

With Fitzpatrick, D. Effects of selective cortical ablation on initiated and elicited sexual behavior in female rats. Western psychological Association, 1969.

With Paloutzian, R. & Moss, R. L. Effects of electrical stimulation of forebrain structures on copulatory behavior of ovariectomized, hormone-treated rats. Western Psychological Association, 1971.

With Spencer, J. D. Behavioral response latencies to intravenous injections of estrogenic and progestational hormones, and the biphasic aspects of progesterone. Western Psychological Association, 1971.

With French, David & Fitzpatrick, D. Sexual preference in the female rat. West Coast Sex Conference, fall, 1971, San Francisco.

With French, David. Copulation in female rats through variation of the ovarian hormones. West Coast Sex Conference, fall, 1971, San Francisco.

With LeGare, Miriam. Responses of single convergent neurons in the basal forebrain of the rat to sexual stimulation. West Coast Sex Conference, fall, 1971, San Francisco.

With LeGare, Miriam. Direct retinal projections to the hypothalamus of the rat. A fiber degeneration study. West Coast Sex Conference, fall, 1971, San Francisco.

With Boerner, Gerald L. Stimulus generalization as a function of brightness and initial preferences. A preliminary analysis of hormone metabolites in brain: Chemical identification. Western Psychological Association, 1972.

With French, David. Participant observation as a patient in a rehabilitation hospital. Western Psychological Association. 1972.

With French, David & LeFare, Miriam. Single unit activity of convergent cells in basal forebrain. Western Psychological Association, 9171.

With LeGare, Miriam. Fiber degeneration studies of direct retino-hypothalamic projections and the implications for behavior. Western Psychological Association, 1972.

With Martin, L.J. The effects of animal odor cues in maze learning. Western Psychological Association, 1972.

With Merlo, Nicholas S. Effects of amygdaloid lesions on the acquisition and extinction of a discriminated operant. Western Psychological Association, 1972.

With Merlo, Nicholas S. The effects of animal odor cues in maze learning. Western Psychological Association, 1972.

With Spencer, James. A preliminary analysis of hormone metabolites in brain: Chemical identification. Western Psychological Association, 1972.

With French, D. & LeGare M. Single unit investigation of multiple modality systems and convergent cells in the hypothalamus. Western Psychological Association, 1972.

With Boerner, Gerald L. & Spencer, James O. A preliminary analysis of hormone metabolites and protein changes in the brain. Rocky Mountain Psychological Association, 1972.

With French, D. J., Leeb, C. S., Fahrion, S. L., & Jecht, E. W. Self-induced scrotal hyperthermia in man followed by decrease in sperm output. A preliminary report. Presented at: West Coast Society for Scientists in the

Study of Sex, (Nov. 12, 1972); Annual Meeting of Biofeedback Research Society, (Nov. 14, 1972): International Conference on Male Contraception, Berlin, Germany, (Dec. 2, 1972); Western Psychological Association, Anaheim, California, (April 12, 1973).

With French, D. J., Leeb, C. S., Fahrion, S. L. & Jecht, E. W. Autogenes Trainin, Scrotum-Temperatur und Spermatozoenzahl. Deutsche Gesellschaft zum Studium der Fertilitat und Sterilitat, Jahres Kongress, April, 1973 in Freiburg (Breisgau).

Sunglass Information. Rudder, January, 1973.

Sound Communication among whales. Rudder, April, 1973 (in press).

With French, D. J., Leeb, C. S., Fahrion, S. L., & Jecht, E. W. Self-induced hyperthermia in man. Journal of biofeedback, 1, #1, 1973, p. 6ff.

With French, D., Leeb, C., Fahrion, S. & Jecht, E. W. Self-induced scrotal hyperthermia in man. Western Psychological Association, 1973.

With Boerner, G. & Gomes M. a unit detection device for use in unrestrained animals: Activity comparisons with normal recording techniques. Western Psychological Association, 1973.

With French, D. J., Leeb, C. S., Fahrion, S.L. Voluntary reversible control of fertility in man via testicular hyperthermia. International Research Communication System, 1973.

Printed in the United States
17397LVS00004B/167